Daily Meditations for Dieters

Daily Meditations for Dieters

How to Think Thin 365 Days a Year

by Anne Colby

A CITADEL PRESS BOOK
Published by Carol Publishing Group

A Citadel Press Book
Published by Carol Publishing Group
Citadel Press is a registered trademark of
    Carol Communications, Inc.
Editorial Offices: 600 Madison Avenue,
    New York, N.Y. 10022
Sales and Distribution Offices: 120
    Enterprise Avenue, Secaucus,
    N.J. 07094
In Canada: Canadian Manda Group, P.O.
    Box 920, Station U, Toronto, Ontario
    M8Z 5P9
Queries regarding rights and permissions
    should be addressed to Carol Publishing
    Group, 600 Madison Avenue, New York,
    N.Y. 10022

Carol Publishing Group books are available at special discounts for bulk purchases,
sales promotion, fund-raising, or educa-
tional purposes. Special editions can be
created to specifications. For details,
contact: Special Sales Department, Carol
Publishing Group, 120 Enterprise Avenue,
Secaucus, N.J. 07094

Manufactured in the United States of
America
10 9 8 7 6 5 4 3 2 1

**Library of Congress Cataloging-in-
Publication Data**
Colby, Anne
    Daily meditations for dieters : how to
    think thin 365 days a year / by Anne
    Colby.
        p.   cm.
        ISBN 0–8065–1580–5
        1. Reducing—Psychological aspects.
    2. Meditations.   I. Title.
    RM222.2.C555   1994
    613.2′5—dc20   94-17784
                                          CIP

Acknowledgments

So many people have supported me in the writing of this book. My thanks first of all to my agent, Susan Urstadt, for her enthusiasm, persistence, and belief in my work. I also want to thank my editors—Jim Ellison, for his infinite patience, graciousness, and good humor; and Eileen Cotton, for seeing the possibilities in the book and agreeing to publish it.

I am grateful to those who have given me friendship and love over the years and provided inspiration. I would especially like to thank Patricia Konley, for her good words and unfailing faith in me; Margot Johnson, for her valuable insights; Kathy Noonan, for her sense of humor and fine example; Sam Greengard, Charlene Marmer Solomon, Tom Johnson, and Robert Massello for their encouragement and seasoned advice; Louise Damberg, Janice Nagano, Bernard Ohanian and Donna Frazier for their professional and personal support; and Beverly Manley Rose, for her wise counsel.

My family is a great source of strength for me, and I am deeply appreciative of their presence in my life. Special thanks to my father and mother, Tom and Carol Colby; to my siblings Tom, Dolly, Dan and Chris Colby; to my grandparents Anne and Carl Oettle, Angela Colby and George Colby; and to my great-aunt and -uncle Anne and Barney Bring.

Preface

My interest in this topic comes from personal experience. I've done battle with the bathroom scales myself. I know that being overweight is the symptom; rarely is it the disease.

I've listened to those who have never had a problem with their weight say, with some measure of judgment, "All you have to do is eat less and you lose weight, right? Isn't that pretty straightforward?" Well, yes and no.

First of all, we are just learning that it is not how much you eat, but what you eat that matters. Whereas once we were advised that bread and potatoes were off-limits to dieters, now we know that butter and oil are the foods that really put on the pounds. We now also know that eating too little can perpetuate the problem and that exercise is important in a reducing program.

Second, few who suffer from being overweight or from eating disorders can resolve their problems by following a diet plan alone. If it were that easy, 33 percent of American adults would not be obese today. No, our relationship with food is much more complex.

This daily meditation book addresses the myriad issues that face those with weight problems and eating disorders. It applies to those who are a mere ten pounds overweight and to those who need to lose much more. It even speaks to those who are underweight or at their ideal weight, yet still torment themselves about their "fat" bodies. It acknowledges that we use food to feed more than our bodies—that we often use it in an attempt to satisfy spiritual, emotional, and intellectual hunger.

Instinctively, all of us know what and how much we need to eat to stay alive and healthy. Unfortunately, those signals are often overwhelmed by a popular culture that alternately teases us with the ready availability of super-sweet and high-fat foods and torments us with media images that encourage us to reduce ourselves to model-thin proportions. Many of us work at jobs that require us to sit for long periods of time; in our fast-is-better world, we speed to our destinations in cars rather than on foot, and rush through meal preparation and enjoyment.

This book provides a first step for those who wish to sort out the conflicting outer signals and reacquaint themselves with their own instincts. It is not a get-thin-fast diet. Rather, it asks readers to gradually adjust their daily habits and examine their attitudes and needs so that they can reach their optimum weight and get off the diet treadmill once and for all.

Daily Meditations for Dieters

JANUARY 1

What is a diet? Something you go on . . . to go off!
—JANE BRODY

D-I-E-T is truly a four-letter word. Over the course of a lifetime, the average dieter loses hundreds of pounds—over and over again. Lately we read about the harmful physical effects from all this dieting. And yet we continue to look for the magic bullet, the quick fix that will take off the ten or twenty-five or fifty pounds by next week. We buy the newest weight-loss book, or join the dieter's club, and then stock our cupboards with the prescribed ammunition: grapefruit, frozen diet dinners, fake food.

Maybe it's time to reconsider.

How about taking the advice of the experts who recommend that you drop the idea of a diet altogether and change your eating habits permanently? It takes time—maybe six months to a year. It takes a change not only in the way you eat, but in the way you live.

Of course, the word *diet* is fine if it's referring to your lifetime eating habits. The important point is that you *change your diet*, not just *go on a diet*. The change doesn't have to be drastic—in fact, it's better if you adjust it a little bit each day. Are you ready to start now?

Since fad diets haven't worked, I'm going to try something new. I will look not only at my eating habits, but at my whole life. Eating for good health begins today.

JANUARY 2

The journey of a thousand miles begins with one step. —LAO-TSU

The first step of any journey is the most important. You can't get anywhere without a beginning. It doesn't even matter what you do.

So forget about starting your diet with a dramatic flourish tomorrow. What small action can you take toward weight reduction right now? You can walk up the two flights of stairs to your office instead of riding the elevator, for one thing. You can substitute nonfat for whole milk in your morning coffee. Small steps like this can start you off on your journey.

I will do whatever I comfortably can right now to begin.

JANUARY 3

What is important is to begin. —HUGH PRATHER

The hardest part is just before you start. That's when fear runs rampant. The resistance to change is immense. The prospect of living the rest of your life without relying on your best friend—food—is overwhelming.

Make it easier for yourself. Don't think of this as a six-week diet or a three-month project, or even something you have to do for the rest of your life. Just stay in the moment. Tell yourself, "Right here, right now, I will eat a balanced meal," and "I will skip the chocolate cake tonight and have a bowl of melon instead." Take each moment as it comes.

Don't think ahead to all the things you will have to give up forever. Just lay the first brick on the foundation. Add one brick at a time and, before you know it, the house will be built.

Nothing ever happens without a beginning. The important thing is to take the first step.

JANUARY 4

You have to have a goal or you're not going anywhere. —BONNIE BLAIR

A goal can be large or small: an important milestone you want to accomplish this year, or a resolution to add more fiber to your diet each day. Goals are helpful to keep you moving forward, rather than running in place.

It's important to set diet goals that are realistic (a twenty-pound loss in two weeks is not). Set goals for the day each morning. Write down your goals for the week, the month, and even the year. Don't just focus on weight loss. Focus on changing your eating habits, too—cutting down on sugar consumption and increasing your intake of fruits and vegetables. And, finally, set goals for other areas of your life. Having a dream that you are working toward will help you let go of your obsession with food.

I will dare to dream and set goals for how I want my life to change.

JANUARY 5

Nothing is particularly hard if you divide it into small jobs. —HENRY FORD

A builder, even though he has the end result in mind, doesn't just tell his workers to construct a house. He assigns jobs in the order in which they must be completed: today the foundation, tomorrow the frame, after that the plumbing, and so on. Day by day, the house goes up.

Any large task, when viewed in its entirety, seems overwhelming. But break it down into small amounts that you can wrap your mind around, and all of a sudden it becomes a manageable project.

View your weight loss in the same way. Take it one pound at a time. Challenge yourself to do the best you can each day.

To reach my goal weight instantly is impossible, but today I can be one step closer.

Becoming an instinctive eater is the key to weight control. —STEVEN C. STRAUSS, M.D., AND GAIL NORTH

What is an instinctive eater? Someone who eats when she's hungry and stops when she's physically satisfied. If you have never allowed yourself to get hungry, or if you've never paid attention to the pattern of your hunger, do it now. Observe how long you can comfortably go without food and how much you need to consume before you are full.

Honoring your body's own hunger signals may mean you eat smaller, more frequent meals to keep your blood sugar on an even keel. Or you may find you do better with only two larger meals a day.

When I eat for reasons besides physical hunger, I will pay attention to when and why.

It is part of the cure to want to be cured.
—SENECA

Desire takes you halfway to success. Your desire to lose weight, feel better, and get in shape will be what carries you to your goal. Without desire there is no spark to begin, no fuel to persevere through hard times.

So bless your restlessness and impatience. Be glad you look in the mirror cursing the way your body looks now. This longing for change is the first step in your journey to better health.

I'm ready to make a positive change.

JANUARY 8

No aim is so high as to justify unworthy methods. —ALBERT EINSTEIN

We are blinded by our goals. We want to lose ten pounds in ten days. We are desperate to fit into a certain dress by spring. We can't bear the thought of wearing a swimsuit, not the way we look now.

And so we starve ourselves (and binge). Eat garbage (and throw up). Consume only diet soda for days (and lose our energy). Have our fat sucked away by liposuction (side effects not yet known). Ruin our health with one fad diet after another.

We've become food-obsessed, and this makes us feel crazy. The ends do not justify the means (and we rarely reach the ends like this, anyway).

Instant results on a drastic weight-loss program are not worth the price of my physical and mental health.

JANUARY 9

Eat your vegetables! —MOM

Mom knew what she was talking about. Vegetables are indeed good for you. The medical and nutritional communities say they should be the foundation of your diet.

When you were a kid, vegetables might have meant all-but-flavorless canned mush or green bits cooked beyond recognition. You came to view them as a necessary evil accompanying the main course. It can be different today.

Buy organic and taste the difference. Shop from small farmers at a farmers' market to see the variety of flavorful vegetables available in season. Sample something you've never tried before. Pick out an old standby you haven't eaten for ages and try it in a new recipe. Make it the center of the meal.

I will make vegetables an important part of my new diet.

Taste the feast by Nature spread.
—SAMUEL JOHNSON

It's easy to be seduced by high-fat and high-sugar fast foods and sweets. It's the rule rather than the exception in our society today. To save the time it takes to cook things ourselves, we consume prepared foods that are loaded with chemicals, calories, and cholesterol. But where is the nourishment that will strengthen us, maintain our immunity against illness, and keep our body's complex systems running properly?

You will go a long way toward making yourself feel better if you eliminate the junk from your diet and rediscover the pleasure of fresh fruits, vegetables, and whole grains. Once you've turned your back on the seduction of processed-sugar products and high-fat snacks, the subtle pleasures of natural foods will emerge. You will begin to appreciate the sublime pleasure of a crisp, sweet apple and slightly bitter leafy greens.

It's time to get rid of the packaged and processed foods. Fill your body with the living nutrients of fruits, vegetables, and nourishing grains—products of soil and sun.

Starting today, I will eat foods from nature that truly nourish my body.

JANUARY 11

Pastry should never be a daily occurrence. When it is rich, it is both good and indigestible; when it is cheap, it is bad and still more indigestible.
—CHRISTINE TERHUNE HERRICK

Is a Paris patisserie your idea of heaven? Or maybe your taste is more along the lines of the local mini-mall donut shop. Either way, the fat and calorie news is not good. But you knew that already!

You've tuned your taste buds to respond enthusiastically to revved-up foods like dense chocolate and butter-rich pastries. The rest of your body does not fare as well. The sugar and fat send your nervous and digestive systems into overdrive.

If you're trying to lose weight, you have two choices. If you trust yourself to stop, you can limit yourself to small portions of these goodies now and then. If you can't stop or if you want to break their hold over you, you probably have to cut them out completely, at least for a while. Make a pact with yourself to stay away from them for at least a month. Tell yourself you can try them again then. After a month of healthful eating, you may find they've become too rich for your taste.

I may be craving rich pastry, but my body certainly doesn't need it.

No great thing is created suddenly, any more than a bunch of grapes or a fig. If you tell me that you desire a fig, I answer that there must be time. Let it first blossom, then bear fruit, then ripen. —EPICTETUS

You may sometimes wish you could snap your fingers and instantly be thin. But as you well know, losing weight and getting into shape take time.

What is really happening during the six weeks or three months or year it takes to reach your desired weight? Your body is using up the fat it has stored from past meals. As you increase your exercise and improve your nutrition, your metabolism is going through changes, speeding up to process food more efficiently. Your muscles are responding to the exercise by toning up and filling out. Your internal organs are adjusting to their new environment. Your body needs this time to adjust.

I can appreciate the complexity of what is happening inside me as my body changes.

If I had two loaves of bread I would sell one to buy a hyacinth to feed my soul.
—ELBERT HUBBARD

Sometimes our hunger is not physical—it's emotional, spiritual, or intellectual. When we mistakenly use food to try to feed one of these other needs, we miss out on an opportunity for real satisfaction. We feed our bodies but starve our souls.

Every time you get an urge to eat today, ask yourself: Am I physically hungry, or would something else satisfy me more than food? Is my stomach empty, or is it my heart, mind, or spirit that needs nourishment instead?

The beauty of nature, a quiet moment, an uplifting experience, and the touch of another person can feed my hunger and nourish my soul.

JANUARY 14

One doesn't discover new lands without consenting to lose sight of the shore for a very long time. —ANDRÉ GIDE

Losing a significant amount of weight means making a big change in your life. It's easy to underestimate that. We think we'll be the same person, only thinner. Not so. If we've done the job properly, at the end of our weight loss it's not just our bodies that will have changed. Our daily habits, our view of the world, and the way we react to events all will have shifted as well.

As we sail away to new places, we can expect to feel somewhat out of sorts. It takes a while to find our sea legs. We must learn to follow our inner compasses as we let go of old ways to reach our new destinations.

I trust my inner compass to guide me safely.

JANUARY 15

It is possible to be so busy going on or off a diet that there isn't time left to enjoy life. —MARCELENE COX

Sometimes we lose perspective. We see ourselves as fat (whether we are or not), and our life revolves around trying to change that. We think about food continually. We weigh our food, drink our diet shakes, obsess about calories, and look into liposuction. We worry about how we look in the mirror, through a camera lens, on the beach, at a dinner party, in bed. In striving to reach our goal—the perfect body—we lose track of the process, which is life. Working, loving, playing, and dreaming is what it's all about.

Today I will take my mind off food and focus on the rest of what life has to offer.

Believe that life is worth living, and your belief will help create the fact. —WILLIAM JAMES

There's a school of psychology that says if you act as if you are confident—or happy or well-adjusted—you eventually will be. Other people treat you as if you were that way, and you treat yourself that way, too. Soon your actions start to drive your beliefs. The change starts on the outside and works its way inside.

How would you behave if you were thin? What would you do differently? Would you eat smaller portions, wear different clothes, relate to other people in another way?

Acting as if you are thin may help you adjust to what life will be like when you have lost weight. And changing "fat" habits to those of a thin person will be instrumental in helping you reach your goal.

I can start living as if I were at my ideal weight right now.

What one has to do usually can be done.
—ELEANOR ROOSEVELT

The word *diet* has lost its meaning because of all our failed attempts. It's come to mean a temporary weight loss, or just a New Year's resolution that's inevitably broken. But it doesn't have to be that way.

You want to change your eating habits permanently, and that's what you're going to do. It's not an impossible task; it's probably not even the hardest thing you've ever had to do. You must only decide that this is what you are committed to, and the rest will fall into place.

I have the strength to stick with it and change my eating habits.

One should seek the company of only such people who call for the exercise of one's good behavior.
—ERNEST VON FEUCHTERSLEBEN

Just as recovering alcoholics often need to stay away from friends who are heavy drinkers (at least during the crucial period before their new habits are established), for awhile you may need to avoid the company of friends who encourage your overeating.

You know the ones. The friend who won't rest until you've ordered the pie à la mode, or a rich chocolate dessert, at the end of a night out. Or the "well-meaning" family members who, when you visit, hound you to eat more—even when you tell them you're full. Or the group whose social activities revolve around gorging on chips and guacamole dip and deep-fried onion rings.

Give them a couple of chances to adjust to your new ways. If they ignore you or belittle your cause, it may be time to rethink the relationship—at least until your new habits are set.

Responsible parents try to keep their children away from bad influences when they're in their care. They know that vices can be tempting. Take care of yourself the same way.

I will surround myself with people who support my new habits.

Sometimes our fate resembles a fruit tree in winter. Who would think at beholding such a sad sight that those jagged twigs will turn green again in the spring and blossom and bear fruit, but we hope it, we know it. —GOETHE

So many things in life we take on faith, and we never even know it. We trust that the trees will return to green in the spring and that we will awaken each morning after we sleep.

In this way, we must also have faith in our own transformations. We see ourselves in our current form and find it hard to believe that life could be any different. But it can. Remarkable changes happen—if not overnight, then in time. If your goal is a new way of eating, a habit of regular exercise, and an improvement in your appearance, it is surely possible that you will see a change by the spring.

Common sense tells you this is possible. What's necessary is the faith to make it so. Let your belief in yourself allow it to happen!

I trust in the possibility of positive change in my life.

The majority of the world's population lives on a more or less vegetarian diet. —KARL BRANDT

Asian cooks use meat as a condiment in their stir-frys and soups, and vegetables often take center stage. Middle- and Near-Eastern cuisines get much of their protein from such foods as lentils, yogurt, and chick-peas. Beans and rice are favored in Mexico and Latin America. And until the twentieth century, meat was served only occasionally, rather than daily in the United States. Today we live in one of the few countries where meat is eaten two or three times a day.

Such quantities of meat as Americans eat may be a sign of affluence, but they're not necessarily a sign of good health. By now we've all heard the warnings about cholesterol and fat intake and protein overload. We know that meat is generally higher in fat than other foods — and harder to digest, as well.

Now is a good time to cut back. Start with a visit to a library or a bookstore to pick up a cookbook with low-fat vegetarian recipes. You'll find a huge variety, covering everything from ethnic cooking to spa cuisine. Try cooking this way for a few weeks, at least. As long as you choose recipes that are low in fat, you will gain new food experiences while you lose weight.

I will keep an open mind as I explore new ways of eating.

One must have something to dream of.
—NIKOLAI LENIN

Before we can successfully make a change, we must be able to envision ourselves doing it. Our dreams are the model for what we eventually become.

Lie back and close your eyes right now. Imagine yourself at your ideal weight. Take yourself on a quick trip through an ordinary day. What do you look like? How do you feel?

Now imagine yourself putting on that dress you've always wanted to wear, finishing the marathon you've always wanted to run, saying no to a rich dessert and not giving it another thought. Take the time to imagine these rewards for your efforts, and remind yourself of them every day.

My dreams will make it so.

Habit is stronger than reason.
—GEORGE SANTAYANA

Your doctor can give you a dozen good reasons to lose weight, but logic only takes you so far. You know you need to lose weight. Doing it is the hard part.

To make it easier, concentrate on improving your exercise and eating habits. It takes just three to four weeks to change them. After a month of regular exercise, working out will be something you do almost without effort. After four weeks of eating naturally low-fat foods, those high in fat will seem abnormally rich.

Once you establish a new routine, willpower becomes less important. The power of habit helps you get to your goal.

I can do anything for a month, including exercising and eating sensibly. After that, it becomes automatic.

Regret is an appalling waste of energy, you can't build on it; it's good only for wallowing in.
— KATHARINE MANSFIELD

It's easy to feel despair over the condition of our bodies if we aren't happy with them. But it's better to pay attention to what our bodies can tell us about the changes we need to make in our lives.

Is your excess weight related to a specific event such as pregnancy or divorce? Maybe you have feelings that still need to be resolved. Has your weight crept up slowly with years of inactivity and bad eating? Perhaps you need to alter your daily habits for a healthier lifestyle. Have you always felt as though you were overweight? Maybe you need to adjust overly harsh attitudes toward yourself and find ways to boost your self-esteem.

What is your body telling you about your life?

I won't turn today into another day of regret by flogging myself for being overweight. I will use it instead to begin building a foundation of better habits.

A man must be strong enough to mold the peculiarity of his imperfections to the perfection of his peculiarities. —WALTER RATHENAU

It's important to trust yourself to figure out what diet and exercise programs are best for you. Different programs work for different people. You want to eventually find a program that will work for the rest of your life.

Some people like clear rules and lots of details about what's allowable and what's not. For those, a preplanned menu and strict exercise regime might be just right. Other people need a program that's a little looser, with just general guidelines about how much fat and how many calories to consume in a day.

A counseling program or twelve-step program might be helpful for some, while others do better with daily meditation. A macrobiotic diet may be perfect for some people, whereas others just want to find ways to stay slim while eating mostly fast foods.

What kind of diet and exercise program complements my life as a whole?

Knowledge is power. —Francis Bacon

Some people are fat not because they eat that much more food, but because what they do eat is loaded with fat. You may be able to lose significant amounts of weight just by watching your consumption of certain high-fat foods.

Recent studies have given us shocking statistics on typical fast-food entrées—hamburgers, Mexican meals, Chinese food—that contain anywhere from thirty-five to ninety-five grams of fat. And this comes when various government and medical reports say we should consume only between fifteen and sixty-five grams of fat a day, depending on our size (and who's doing the study).

We've learned to pay attention to how many calories are contained in different foods. Now it's time to become aware of how much fat there is in the foods we eat, too.

I can reduce just by learning to look for fat content on the nutritional labels.

To blind oneself to change is not therefore to halt it. —Isaac Goldberg

Has your weight slowly crept up higher and higher? Does it feel like your life has started to slip out of control? Your impulse may be to ignore it. "I will deal with it tomorrow," you say. "After all, I'm not that heavy. So I'm not happy. Who is?"

It's your business if you want to put things off and avoid looking at your life. But at least admit to yourself that this is what you are doing. When things are wrong, they stay wrong until you make a change. Precisely when you choose to do that is up to you alone.

Hiding my head in the sand doesn't change things. It only buys me extra time.

We cannot do everything at once, but we can do something at once. —CALVIN COOLIDGE

If getting started is the hardest thing, then sticking with our program when we haven't yet seen significant results runs a close second.

It takes faith to believe we can make it, hope to keep us going, and love to tell us that we deserve to get there. We're not going to reach our goals tomorrow, or even next week. But each little action you take today—ordering a lightly dressed salad instead of a steak, taking a swim when you feel like snacking—brings you that much closer. How much better to do something today and be thinner in six months than to give up altogether and never reach our goals.

Each tiny gesture is significant in the bigger picture.

There are some remedies worse than the disease. —PUBLILIUS SYRUS

Syrus must have been thinking about the five-hundred-calorie-a-day diets some of us resort to in an effort to lose extra weight fast. These are remedies in name only. In reality, extreme calorie-cutting is one of the worst ways to lose (and keep off) the pounds. When we resort to starvation-level eating, our metabolism slows down to keep us alive. We don't lose fat, we lose water weight, which quickly returns when we start eating again. Worse, our skin, hair, and disposition all suffer. This kind of diet is a disease, not a solution. If it's a constant temptation for you, seek professional help.

Food obsession can show itself in eating too little, as well as in eating too much.

JANUARY 29

Still round the corner there may wait, a new road, or a secret gate. —J. R. R. TOLKIEN

When we were little, everything was a new experience. We were discovering things for the first time, so life was filled with surprise. But as we got older, we learned what to expect from our normal routines. We lost our sense of wonder.

We can go back and cultivate what one Zen Buddhist master calls "beginner's mind." This is the ability to approach the world without preconceptions. As we open ourselves to the possibility of new experiences, we find they almost magically appear: new people, new places, new ideas we've never considered before.

If I keep my eyes open, I may stumble upon that secret gate.

JANUARY 30

Have patience with all things, but chiefly have patience with yourself. Do not lose courage in considering your own imperfections, but instantly set about remedying them—every day begin the task anew. —ST. FRANCIS DE SALES

It takes patience to continue day by day through the seemingly endless task of eliminating bad habits and then waiting for the reward—weight loss—to appear. Then one night we go out to eat with friends and get carried away; the results show up on the scale the next day. (Why does it seem to take so long to lose weight but not the other way around?) If our resolve is low, we may come close to giving up altogether.

But we won't give up. We are committed to losing weight. A weight gain is disappointing, but it's only a temporary setback in a lifelong process. We will carry on.

I will never go wrong as long as I look for the lessons in everything I do.

Talents are best nurtured in solitude; character is formed in the stormy billows of the world.
— GOETHE

Reading all the self-help books in the world is useless if we're too scared to get out there and live. Certainly there is value in reflection and private study. Many areas of our personalities are best developed on our own.

But to shape the raw material of our characters, we must expose ourselves to the bumps and sharp edges and rocky paths of life. Interacting with other people, trying our best, making mistakes, and learning each lesson is the hard work of being human. But what satisfaction we have at the end of the day!

I look for the lesson in all of life's experiences.

$\mathscr{F}$EBRUARY 1

Your daily life is your temple and your religion.
—Kahlil Gibran

When we abuse our bodies by starving and bingeing, we commit a crime against ourselves and against God. We were given bodies with designs that come close to perfection. Think of the miracle being performed right now: hearts, lungs, eyes, minds—every part of us—working together in a complex harmony. Every aspect of life is a miracle unfolding before our eyes. How ungrateful of us to fail to appreciate this amazing gift.

I can show my appreciation in the simple act of living well.

FEBRUARY 2

All happiness depends on a leisurely breakfast.
— JOHN GUNTHER

Sometimes it really is this simple. Breakfast may or may not be the time when you are hungriest, but nutritionists agree that a good breakfast helps control overeating during the rest of the day. Include fruit, grains and other energy-boosting foods.

Start the day early, giving yourself enough time for a leisurely, enjoyable meal. This will set the tone for the day.

By taking time for myself first thing in the morning, I will have more to offer others later in the day.

FEBRUARY 3

There is nothing wrong with making mistakes. Just don't respond with encores.
— ANONYMOUS

Yikes! You've eaten the whole plateful of fries, scarfed down the tray of cookies, or inhaled a family-size portion of cheese lasagna. Yes, you've blown it. But what will you do next?

One approach is to declare everything else in the refrigerator fair game, since you've already come this far. Not a good move! A better response would be to savor the food you've eaten (after all, the damage is already done), walk away from the disaster site, and put it behind you. Then schedule an extra exercise session to burn off some of those calories.

Everybody, myself included, makes mistakes. I live with my imperfections and learn from them.

FEBRUARY 4

Life on the farm is a school of patience: you can't hurry the crops or make an ox in two days.
—HENRI FOURNIER ALAIN

One of the things that's so difficult about weight loss is that it takes so long. As much as you may want to be thin *now*, that's just physically impossible. You can fool yourself with pronouncements about dropping two dress sizes in as many weeks, but—short of going on a total fast —you just ain't gonna get there that quickly.

So why not relax and enjoy the ride? Congratulate yourself as you keep up your daily walks or workouts. Pay attention to how your body is toning up and how once-tight clothes are starting to fit more comfortably. Notice when your cravings for sweets or junk food become less pronounced or disappear.

Since I can't get to my goal instantly, I'll take time to enjoy the process.

FEBRUARY 5

Every minute starts an hour.
—PAUL GONDOLA

This statement is a good antidote to the all-or-nothing thinking that is common among dieters. "I ate three cookies, so I might as well eat the whole box." "I missed two days of exercise, so what's the use of continuing it at all?" "I gained back a pound, so I might as well eat whatever I want because the rest are sure to follow."

Don't wait until tomorrow to start over. Start now. Each minute brings an opportunity to begin again.

Forget the mistakes I made yesterday or this morning, I will begin again this minute.

Before everything else, getting ready is the secret of success. —HENRY FORD

Do you think you will magically become a new person on the day you reach your goal weight? If so, you are in for a rude shock. If you haven't already examined your attitudes and beliefs and altered bad habits, you will find yourself the same person you were before, but minus X number of pounds. And then, because nothing but the externals have changed, the excess weight is more likely to return.

For example, a layer of fat can be protection for some people—from sexuality, or from a perceived threat in the environment. If this is true for you, counseling or a therapy group might be helpful, so that you don't feel defenseless when you lose that fat. Others are saddled with a lack of self-worth that, if not dealt with, will still be there when they're swathed in a size six. You may be able to lose weight without understanding why you gained it in the first place, but you probably won't be able to keep it off for the rest of your life.

I will prepare myself for the success that is coming.

Less is more. —MIES VAN DER ROHE

As you cut down on fat and refined sugar in your diet, your taste for them will lessen. As you reduce the amount of food you eat, your desire for excessive amounts will eventually go away. Whole milk will taste as rich as cream. Fresh fruit will seem intensely sweet, and vegetables more flavorful than you could have ever imagined. Candy and other manufactured sweets will start to taste overdone. Meals you easily consumed at one sitting will now provide enough food for the whole day.

Less will become more as I improve my eating habits.

Never cut what you can untie.
—JOSEPH JOUBERT

Weight that comes off more slowly stays off longer. That's the official decree from the diet establishment.

Why? It's more than just a matter of it being better to slowly change your habits and get used to a new lifestyle, although that is a big part of it. There are also biological reasons why you should take it slow. If you cut off your food supply too radically, your body goes into starvation mode and slows your metabolism so you burn fewer calories. When your diet is over and your calorie intake goes back up, your metabolism continues to burn at the same low rate.

Losing a little weight at a time is better than taking it off all at once.

Probably the most satisfying soup in the world for people who are hungry, as well as for those who are tired or worried or cross or in debt or in a moderate amount of pain or in love or in robust health or in any kind of business huggermuggery is minestrone. —M. F. K. FISHER

Let's face it. Food offers more to us than just vitamins and fiber and protein. Some foods make us feel warm and cozy on a rainy day. Others are what we crave when we're in love. And when we're feeling out of sorts with the world, a nourishing soup may be just what we need to stave off our hunger, strengthen our bodies, and fill our bellies. A good minestrone contains very little fat, but lots of nutritional foods: broth, beans, potatoes, pasta, onions, garlic, tomatoes, carrots, and any other vegetables we want to throw in. If you're looking for a comforting food to salve an emotional ill, turn first to those—such as minestrone—with good nutrition to offer as well.

When I need nourishment, I will turn to foods that truly offer it.

And it is well to eat slowly: The food seems to be more plentiful, probably because it lasts longer.
—M. F. K. FISHER

Each time you find yourself wolfing down a meal, stop! When you gulp down your food you will feel you haven't eaten at all. So take a few deep breaths and slow down. Enjoy the meal, bite by bite. Sample each dish as if you were a gourmet. Savor the individual flavors, aromas, and textures. Make the food last longer, and you will find you need to eat less of it.

I will take the time to appreciate food as I eat it, rather than anticipate the next bite.

We have met the enemy, and he is us.
—WALT KELLY

Are you your own best friend or worst enemy? If you aren't sure, start paying attention to the voice that plays inside your head. Does it offer support and encouragement, or "I told you so's" and other disparaging comments?

You may find your inner critic is doing more harm than good. Continue to pay attention to what it's saying and start to rewrite the script. When the voice says, "You can't do that," counter it with "I can." When anxiety overtakes you, treat yourself gently, as you would a dear friend. You don't have to be hard on yourself to ensure that you'll keep trying. In fact, you'll probably find that treating yourself with kindness is what brings out your best.

I will be kind to myself today.

What I love most is an abundance of simple food of perfect quality and staggering freshness, very simply and respectfully treated, tasting strongly of itself. —SYBILLE BEDFORD

Since you are beginning to build your diet on fruits, vegetables, and grains, it makes sense to choose the highest quality and most flavorful items you can buy. Can't afford it, you say? Not so.

You're already saving money by cutting out fast-food meals, over-processed snacks, and packaged desserts, and cutting back on the amount of meat you consume. Why not spend those savings on a snack of organically grown baby carrots, which are sweeter and tastier than the ordinary supermarket variety, or a special-occasion fruit such as blueberries or mangos for dessert?

By "treating" yourself to the best of the healthful foods, you won't feel deprived. The temptation to fill up on junk food will be less. And you will soon find that you enjoy the natural flavor of fresh foods much more.

Rather than skimp, I'll look for the highest quality fresh and whole foods when I shop.

A cynic is not merely one who reads bitter lessons from the past, he is one who is prematurely disappointed in the future. —SIDNEY HARRIS

Never and *always* are much-used words in the cynic's vocabulary. "Things will never change" and "I always do this" are typical litanies of the disappointed dieter who has lost hope in her ability to shape the future.

Do you treat your mistakes as failures that confirm your low self-image? Have you defeated yourself before you've even started?

Just because you were overweight as a child does not mean you will be so for the rest of your life. Just because you overate last night does not mean you have to do so in the future.

Start small. Keep a promise to yourself in this moment. Extend it another moment. And again. If you lapse, see what you can learn from that, and keep going. This time you won't be starting from zero, you'll be building from a foundation of small successes. You will slowly repair your faith in yourself.

I will keep an open mind about the future.

It is one thing to be moved by events; it is another to be mastered by them.
—RALPH W. SOCKMAN

Who among us has ever been completely satisfied with his or her lot in life? Some of us were not given the childhood we would have wanted. Or we wish we had gotten a better education, or had made a different decision about our careers. And our bodies—well, the popularity of plastic surgery and fad diets attests to the fact that few are ever happy with those.

The only thing we can do about the parts of our lives that are truly out of our control is to say, "Oh, well," and carry on. Sighing about what never was may be useful in therapy, but at some point it becomes meaningless. Life didn't deal you a perfect deck of cards. Join the crowd.

But who knows what amazing things you can accomplish with what you were given? The only way to find out is to begin to live, right here, right now.

I will accept the past as a given and do what I can today.

Saying no thank you is still the best reducing exercise. —JOHN NEWTON BAKER

Practice saying no from time to time when food is offered you, especially when you are not hungry and would be accepting it just to be polite. If you are a guest in someone's home, and they insist, ask for a glass of ice water or a cup of tea instead. Often the host is just trying to be gracious.

If the dish being served is something you love—and yet you know you're not really hungry—tell yourself that today is not the last time it will be available. There will be plenty of times to sample it later, when you have an appetite or perhaps when you have lost your irrational craving for it.

And don't feel you have to offer any explanation, unless you want to discuss your weight-reduction program to get their support. Gratuitously announcing that you're on a diet makes everyone else feel self-conscious about their own consumption and adds nothing of interest to social conversation.

I don't have to eat everything that is put before me. I will say no today, knowing the food will still be there another time.

Another good reducing exercise consists in placing both hands against the table edge and pushing back. —ALEXANDER WOOLLCOTT

Your meal's over, and here comes the waiter with the dessert cart. Don't torment yourself. Before the tour of luscious-looking temptations begins, ask for decaf coffee or tea instead. Or, better yet, suggest to your companion that you continue your conversation with a leisurely walk around the block.

The same applies at home. After you've eaten your meal, get up from the table and clear the dishes. Don't allow yourself to continue nibbling on food you don't really need. The time to stop is just before you feel full.

I will remove myself physically from the source of temptation rather than test my resolve by lingering at the table.

Faith is love of the invisible, trust in the impossible, in the improbable. —GOETHE

We look in the mirror and see a fat person. We look into the past, and a chubby child emerges in the fog of our memories. Have we always been fat, or is that just the way we remember it now? And if we've always carried this extra weight, is it possible we will ever lose it? What will our lives be like then?

Faith is what so many of us don't have, and what we need most right now. It's difficult to believe that something we can't see—something we've perhaps never seen—could actually come true.

Release your preconceived ideas of who you are. Let your imagination soar. What will you look like at your ideal weight? What will you wear? How will you relate to other people? What will your typical day be like?

Faith will carry me through the sea of self-doubts.

FEBRUARY 18

A man should not strive to eliminate his complexes, but to get into accord with them; they are legitimately what directs his conduct in the world. —SIGMUND FREUD

If you're getting rid of junk food in your diet, you can work with your cravings instead of fighting them. Buy low-fat foods that mimic the sensations you are seeking.

If you are a nervous eater who often snacks on crunchy chips, keep a bag of mini rice cakes or raw sugar snap peas at hand. If it's something smooth and creamy you are after when you head for the ice cream carton, substitute nonfat yogurt—frozen or refrigerated. And so on. Keep in mind the timing of your eating patterns. Don't be caught off guard by mid-afternoon or late-night food cravings.

If I know my eating habits and food cravings, I can work with them.

FEBRUARY 19

When written in Chinese, the word crisis is composed of two characters. One represents danger, and the other represents opportunity.
—JOHN F. KENNEDY

You've probably heard it before: Adversities are opportunities. They can open the doors to change. If these doors keep popping up in your face, it probably means you're ready to walk through. Life is presenting you with a chance to reach a resolution. A turning point will take you to a new place.

How will I react to the next crisis in my life? Will I turn it into an opportunity?

Life, as it is called, is for most of us one long postponement. —HENRY MILLER

It is easy to fall into the trap of postponing our lives until after we have lost unwanted weight. We are self-conscious about the way we look, so we tell ourselves we'll wait until we can present our slim selves to people, later. We put off exercising because we don't want to be seen in workout clothes, struggling and out of breath. Or maybe we've just gotten into the habit of thinking that life will begin "tomorrow."

Sit down for a few minutes and make a list of the hobbies or activities you've always wanted to pursue. Then stop and consider each one. Is there a good reason you shouldn't do this now? Or is there a way you could try it without making a huge commitment? You could go to one "tryout" dance class, for example, and see how you like it. The hardest part is just getting there.

I will stop postponing my dreams and begin to live them.

While I am busy with little things, I am not required to do greater things.
—St. Francis de Sales

We set ourselves up for failure by taking on too big a task. There's nothing wrong with setting goals, but to sit down to each meal with the thought, "I have to lose thirty pounds so I'd better be good," can be overwhelming. It's tempting to give up when the goal seems so far away.

Rather, take it one step at a time. Little by little, change your approach to food and eating. Spend a bit of extra time at the supermarket reading labels for fat content and calories. Research restaurants in your neighborhood that offer low- or no-fat cooking (some will make up special dishes if you ask). Begin each meal with the resolution that you will eat for both enjoyment and good health.

Weight loss will come as I gradually improve my relationship with food.

Fate shuffles the cards and we play.
—Arthur Schopenhauer

Eating disorders often start in childhood, for food intake is the one thing children can control when everything else is beyond their power. If they have not been given the tools to deal with overwhelming events or emotions, children may turn to food. They can use food to either comfort or punish themselves for perceived wrongs. They may eat or refrain from eating to manipulate others and give themselves a sense of control.

Even if we learned to use food to cope with life's difficulties when we were children, it's not too late now to teach ourselves new tricks. We can relearn ways to play the hands we're given, using healthier strategies to stay in the game.

No one has control over events, but we can choose how we respond to them.

The harder you work, the luckier you get.
— GARY PLAYER

Some people have all the luck, right? Well, sort of. But that's not the whole story.

What looks like luck is usually a blend of other ingredients: working hard, listening to intuition, cultivating a social network, being open to new ideas, exploring opportunities, getting out there, always trying, and persevering. When people explain away other people's good fortune as "luck," it's because they don't see the preparation that went into the final product. "Lucky" people spend more time preparing for positive changes than they do worrying aloud about what could go wrong.

I will invite luck into my life through thoughtful preparation.

When you laugh, laugh like hell, and when you get angry, get good and angry. Try to be alive. You will be dead soon enough.
— WILLIAM SAROYAN

We live in a Prozac world. We are afraid to feel. So we take a pill to regulate and modulate and keep our emotions within bounds.

"Anger is scary — don't show it." "Joy is so corny — stay cool instead." "The workplace is too serious for laughter — be safe and don't take any chances."

How confining to live this way! To live enthusiastically is to live fully. When you feel things, really feel them. Don't try to mask them, don't try to hide. The edges are the boundaries that define the middle ground. Without them life is just an endless, boring plateau.

Emotions give my life shape and color.

One must eat to live, not live to eat.
— MOLIÈRE

Much of what is on supermarket shelves today offers virtually nothing nutritious for our bodies. Many food products offer little more than empty calories and palate-pleasing sensations. They stoke our desire to consume more than we really need because they don't give us anything that is truly satisfying.

Make it your aim to break the sugar habit, cut back on fats, and eat whole foods that nourish your body. Eat real food—don't settle for poor substitutes. When you get back to healthy eating, you will naturally and easily drop down to a healthy weight for your body and build.

The purpose of eating is to sustain life. I will consume only as much as I need.

He who laughs, lasts.
— MARY PETTIBONE POOLE

Even during the "serious" business of dieting, take time to laugh. In fact, laugh even more when engaged in serious pursuits! It makes the dreariness of goal-oriented activities so much more bearable.

Health professionals say humor lengthens our life spans. But no matter if we live to one hundred or not, laughter improves the quality of our lives while we are here.

I will find every occasion to have a good laugh today.

Many a man who would not dream of putting too much pressure in his automobile tires lays a constant overstrain on his heart and arteries.
—BRUCE BARTON

When you regularly consume large quantities of fat, alcohol, sugar, and salt, you are placing a great stress on your body. All of these foods tax both the organs and the glands responsible for processing them. A lifetime of abuse creates predictable results: heart disease, diabetes, liver failure, gallstones—the list goes on.

For good health, nutritionists recommend a diet high in complex carbohydrates (which are easy to digest) and low in processed sugar, salt, and fat. Doesn't this make sense?

I will maintain my body properly by giving it the fuel it needs to run well.

Life consists not simply in what heredity and environment do to us but in what we make out of what they do to us.

—HARRY EMERSON FOSDICK

Your mother has heavy thighs and, lucky you, you got them, too. Your dad has a cholesterol count in the upper ranges, and the doctor says yours is right up there, too. You grew up eating fried everything. Klutz is your middle name.

Even if obesity and lack of coordination run in your family, be glad there isn't something worse. Fat you can do something about. Exercise is within your control. Whatever the story of your family's past, you can still do the best you can with whatever you've been "blessed" with—today.

I don't have to be perfect. I can do a lot if I only try.

MARCH 1

To eat is a necessity, but to eat intelligently is an art.
—LA ROCHEFOUCAULD

Do you know specifically what you should and should not be eating to lose weight? A lot of dieters go wrong because they severely restrict their food intake. They eventually tire of being hungry and give up in discouragement. Yet the latest nutritional advice prescribes an all-you-can-comfortably-eat diet of foods that are very low in fat and processed sugar. If you don't know exactly what this means, pay a visit to your local bookstore or library and read the latest literature. Study the charts that tell how much fat is contained in each food, so you know beforehand what that handful of peanuts on the airplane is going to do to your fat intake for the day.

I will take the time to educate myself about nutrition and food values.

MARCH 2

To every thing there is a season, and a time to every purpose under the heaven.
— ECCLESIASTES 3:1

Change may seem frightening at times, but it is a natural process. It is only when we stand in its way that we get into trouble. The key is to live in the present and stay true to our instincts.

Nature is a wonderful teacher of this lesson. We need only to look outside to observe a million perfect models for change: every plant in the ground, every animal we can see. We, too, are part of the ever-evolving cycle of life. We only need to give in and let it take us along.

I trust in the process of life.

MARCH 3

We accept the verdict of the past until the need for change cries out loudly enough to force upon us a choice between the comforts of further inertia and the irksomeness of action.
— LEARNED HAND

You've decided it's time to let go of your food obsession. In the past it served as protection for you, was a substitute for love, or just reflected a carelessness you had about yourself. But something has changed. No longer are these payoffs enough to compensate for the bad way you feel about yourself when you binge, the limits on your physical prowess because of your extra weight, or the reduced lifespan that could be in the cards if you don't change. As difficult as change always is, you've decided it's worth the trouble.

When I am tempted to turn back, I will remember I am making this change for a good reason. I wasn't happy with the way things were in my life before.

MARCH 4

Forgiveness is the finding again of a lost possession—hatred an extended suicide.
—FRIEDRICH SCHILLER

Hating our bodies (and ourselves) for the shape we are in is one of the worst crimes we can commit against ourselves. As long as we view our body as the enemy, we are trapped in a jail of our own making. When we are unable to love ourselves freely and unconditionally, we have sentenced ourselves to a slow death, wasting away the gift that was handed to us at birth.

Freedom comes only with forgiveness. We start by forgiving ourselves. Our pardon extends to others around us to whom we've assigned blame.

Hatred snuffs out the life we were given. Only forgiveness brings it back.

MARCH 5

We too, the children of earth, have our moon phases all through any year; the darkness, the delivery from darkness, the waxing and waning. None lives, except the mindless, who does not in some degree experience this. —FAITH BALDWIN

If only I could be dumb and happy, we think in our more desperate moments. But we aren't; we have minds and emotions and spirits that perceive the complexities of the world, its heartaches as well as its beauty. When we feel pain, or sadness, we are only reacting thoughtfully to experiences that cross our path.

Don't wish for mindlessness. Don't reach for pills or pastry to drown out your sorrows. Be happy to feel things strongly—a sign that you are truly alive.

Dark emotions, like phases of the moon, pass through my life. I will not hang onto them, nor will I block their arrival.

Happiness is essentially a state of going somewhere, wholeheartedly, one-directionally, without regret or reservation. —WILLIAM H. SHELDON

When you decide to do something, whether it be losing weight or becoming a world-class skater, commit yourself to it. It's always easy to second-guess ourselves, and wonder if we should do something else instead. But give yourself a chance to really succeed. Keep your eyes focused on your desire and learn to block out distractions.

Saying yes to one thing means saying no to a thousand others.

Things forbidden have a secret charm.
—TACITUS

You know what happens when you tell a child not to touch a stove. Or when you forbid your teenager to see certain friends. They may not have really wanted to do it before but, boy, do they want to now! Their attraction to that which is prohibited grows that much stronger.

The same thing happens to you when you set up certain foods as "off-limits": They take on a certain allure. Making foods you like verboten gives them unnecessary power in your life.

My food cravings will only become worse if I set up all-or-nothing scenarios. I will find the middle way.

MARCH 8

It's all right to drink like a fish if you drink what a fish drinks. —MARY PETTIBONE POOLE

For some people who are overweight, the problem lies not in what they are eating, but in what they are drinking. If you suspect that you may be putting down a few too many drinks—even if only from time to time—it might be wise to take yourself to a meeting of Alcoholics Anonymous or to a counselor to discuss it. Don't wait until it makes a disaster of your life. Do something now.

If alcohol is a problem in my life, I will come clean about it.

MARCH 9

Bad habits are trying to call our attention to some part of our lives that is unlived or unexpressed. —SIDRA STONE

Scratch the surface of an overeating habit and you will often find a dream that is being deferred. What is your dream? What challenge are you avoiding by staying fat? What is your excess weight trying to tell you?

It's helpful to ask ourselves these questions, and then write out our answers on paper. Some may benefit additionally from a conversation with a counselor or close friend. Investigate your own psyche as if you were a detective trying to solve a mystery. In unlocking the clues, you will discover your own life's potential.

My life does not start tomorrow; it is being lived today.

A man must learn to forgive himself.
—ARTHUR DAVISON FICKE

As long as you harbor animosity toward yourself, you will continue to neglect or abuse yourself in some way. It may be with food, or drugs, or bad relationships. It all adds up to the same thing: self-hate.

What could you possibly have done that can't be forgiven? How much time have you wasted in anger toward yourself since that time?

I, like all other creatures, am worthy of love.

Happiness comes of the capacity to feel deeply, to enjoy simply, to think freely, to risk life, to be needed. —STORM JAMESON

There are a million recipes for the good life inscribed in ancient religious texts and modern anthologies. Though they vary in the specifics, they agree on some general themes: Live simply and don't put your faith in material things; give and you will receive; trust in a higher power than yourself.

What is your recipe for happiness? Take a few minutes to write it down. Now imagine that you have all of the ingredients at hand. Are you any happier?

Maybe I already possess the things that will make me happy.

When things come to the worst, they generally mend. —SUSANNA MOODIE

At some point you may become discouraged about how slowly the pounds are coming off. No matter how well you are eating and exercising, the weight loss seems to stall, or even halt completely, from time to time.

This is a well-documented occurrence in the course of weight loss. But if you keep going and don't abandon your weight-loss program, this plateau phase will only be temporary, and the pounds will continue to drop off eventually.

Bolster your spirits by staying off the scales for awhile and finding other sources of motivation. Buy a new cookbook with low-fat gourmet recipes and cook a few for your friends. Take up a new sport, such as rock-climbing or Rollerblading, where the point is to have fun. Above all, keep going. Things will improve.

Even though it seems at times that nothing gets any better, I have faith that my situation will improve.

If Winter comes, can Spring be far behind?
—SHELLEY

Every year, nature reminds us that the longest, darkest days are a prelude to the season of growth and rebirth. All living things rest and regenerate during the cold and fallow days of winter to prepare for spring's arrival.

When you reach those dark periods when progress seems to come to a halt, remember that such times are only part of the cycle of change. It only seems as though nothing is happening. When this phase passes—and it's going to—you will look back in wonder at the amazing changes that occurred almost imperceptibly right under your nose.

We need fallow periods in order to absorb change and let our new habits take root.

If one advances confidently in the direction of his dreams, and endeavours to live the life which he has imagined, he will meet with a success unexpected in common hours.
—HENRY DAVID THOREAU

Within each one of us is an inner guide that will lead us safely down the path of life. We need only listen to our instincts, pay attention to our intuition, and imagine for ourselves the life we want to live. When we do, we find that our days have become so much easier. Doors open to us. Setbacks do not stun us but seem to have a rightful place in the scenario. Our inner and outer selves merge to become one. What once were just dreams become our reality.

I will listen to my inner guide as I follow my dreams to the place I have imagined.

It is not easy to find happiness in ourselves and it is not possible to find it elsewhere.
—AGNES REPPLIER

We are given numerous reasons to be unhappy with ourselves every time we pick up a magazine or turn on the TV. The message is painfully clear: Our bodies are not thin enough, our breasts are not large enough, our smiles are not bright enough, our skin is not clear enough, our personalities are not winning enough.

It takes courage to ignore the propaganda and turn away. But that's what we must do.

As long as we search outside ourselves for validation, we will be slaves to changing fashions and to those who have an interest in keeping us in a state of discontent.

I know best what is right for me.

Worry never robs tomorrow of its sorrow; it only saps today of its strength. —A. J. CRONIN

People who worry a lot always think they have good reason to do so. Every misfortune they encounter only proves to them that they were right in anticipating the worst that can happen.

But worry never heads off trouble in advance, as they seem to believe. It only takes away the peace of mind they might have today.

Save your strength for dealing with real adversity when it finally arrives. Worrying only wastes precious time that could be saved for the good experiences waiting for you today.

I do not anticipate misfortune and pain, but let life happen as it will.

It is not immoral not to finish a meal, but it is of questionable morality to treat yourself like a waste-disposal system. —JANE BRODY

Do you remember, as a child, trying to leave the dinner table before finishing everything on your plate? Were you told to "think of the starving children in (impoverished country of your choice)"? Perhaps the message was "You're not leaving until you clean your plate."

It's hard to let go of such thoughts because they are so ingrained. Realistically, we know that a few bites wasted don't create a national garbage crisis. Nor will these bites impoverish our families. But they will, if habitually consumed when we have already eaten enough, slowly add up to extra unneeded pounds.

I will treat my body well by eating only what I truly need and want.

If at first you don't succeed, you're running about average. —M. H. ALDERSON

Often we are harder on ourselves than we are on anyone else. If a friend were struggling to break a bad habit, you would probably offer encouragement and tell her not to be too hard on herself. Why? Because you know it's only human to try, fail, try again, and eventually succeed.

Give yourself the same kind of care and understanding you give to other people. So you slip up now and then—what's new? You aren't perfect! (Who would want to be?) Allow yourself to be the human being that you are.

I will be patient with myself today.

MARCH 19

Balance the day, not each meal in the day.
—M. F. K. FISHER

While being conscious of what you eat is important, there's no need to be obsessive about the subject. Yes, you should eat several servings of fruit, vegetables, and grains each day—but you don't necessarily have to eat them all in the same meal.

You know your own needs and cravings better than anyone else. If you're not a big breakfast eater, perhaps a bowl of fruit and a plain bagel are all you want to eat in the morning. Lunchtime could be grilled meat and a vegetable or an order of sushi; and dinner, a big salad.

Some people feel better with a neat combination of food groups at every meal—but if you're not like them, don't worry. Our bodies still operate as though we were hunter-gatherers on the plains. Foods were eaten as we found them—wild greens here, an occasional animal kill there. As long as we keep to a generally nutritious plan for each day, we can still eat pretty much as though we lived in more primitive (and, food-wise, more healthy) times.

I balance my nutrition throughout the day, according to my body's own needs.

MARCH 20

All desire is a prophecy.
— FATHER VINCENT MCNABB

The act of thinking about our goals and then writing them down on paper can be a powerful step toward achieving them. When we verbalize what we want and then commit our goals to paper, we activate them. Even if we put that sheet away in a drawer, the ideas have been planted in our minds; they now exist as a thought. From that thought comes our actions, now focused in a beneficial direction.

Our desire helps bring our dreams to life.

MARCH 21

Monotony is the awful reward of the careful.
— A. G. BUCKHAM

Don't let your diet and exercise program settle into a humdrum routine—keep them varied and alive! When you get bored with aerobics, switch to a rowing machine for awhile. Alternate swimming and step classes within the same week. Keep your menus interesting. Try out a new restaurant or take-out place every couple of weeks. Give yourself rewards on a regular basis.

Don't let yourself be tempted to abandon your program just to add excitement to your life. Add some spice to your diet right now.

I am creating a diet and exercise program for a lifetime. It can be as interesting as I want to make it.

Nothing will strengthen a man more than the confidence shown in him. —GOETHE

No one can accomplish goals alone. If you haven't yet, now is the time to draw on others for support in your endeavor. A friend's positive attitude can keep you going when you reach a low point. Your husband or companion may be happy to offer support when you need it. And your children may be helpful in encouraging good health habits.

Sometimes all you need to hear is, "You're doing fine. I know you can do it. Remember, it takes time."

Don't wait for people to give you the good words; ask for them. Tell someone you trust that you need encouragement right now, and usually he or she will respond positively. If this doesn't work, try someone else. And if you feel you have no one to turn to for support, seek it out from a group designed to provide it. Almost every community has a Weight Watchers or Overeaters Anonymous support group.

I will learn to seek the help of others to support me in my goals.

No man's life, even the happiest, is without its struggles and sacrifices, for genuine happiness comes to each of us only insofar as our emotions make us independent of fate.
—WILHELM VON HUMBOLDT

When we are young, our happiness depends on things beyond our control. We wonder whether the boy we are enamored of likes us. We worry about whether we are popular with our friends. We hope we will be accepted into the college of our choice, or find a job.

It's possible to be consumed with these kinds of matters until we die. Disappointments bring heartache and self-pity, or anger and resentment. Achievements result in elation and joy. The roller coaster of life continues.

One of the benefits of growing older is seeing how our happiness and self-esteem can be independent of outside events. Your best friend may shun you, creditors may threaten, your boss may not realize your worth, but your belief in your own self-worth need not be harmed.

My self-esteem does not depend on the event of the moment. The scenery changes, but my worth remains the same.

More die in the United States of too much food that of too little. —J. K. GALBRAITH

We are one of the most prosperous societies in the world and one that is blessed with a vast selection of reasonably priced food. Because of this, we have grown used to consuming large amounts of it. We eat much more than we need—more than is good for us. Too, many still operate under the mistaken belief that our bodies need animal protein at each meal. This kind of diet does more harm than good, often resulting in high blood pressure and heart attacks.

Don't strain your system by forcing it to digest large quantities of fat and protein. If you feel bloated or sick when you leave the table, you've eaten too much. Eat lightly and give your body a rest.

I'm better off eating a little less rather than a little more.

As for me, except for an occasional heart attack, I feel as young as I ever did.
—ROBERT BENCHLEY

When we're young, we take our health for granted, but as we grow older we accumulate aches and injuries. Pretty soon our medicine cabinets are stocked with pills. We believe this is the way it's supposed to be.

But what if it isn't? What if headaches and heart attacks and hemorrhoids could be headed off by good nutrition, exercise, and stress management? We're learning that this often can be the case.

What does your medicine cabinet look like? Are you only treating the symptoms of diseases when you could prevent them completely by taking better care of your health?

I will pay attention to how my daily habits affect the condition of my health.

A man hath no better thing under the sun, than to eat, and to drink, and to be merry.
— ECCLESIASTES 8:15

In your enthusiasm for losing weight, it's important not to get carried away. Don't dine like a pauper at every meal; take time to sup like a king now and then, too! Remember how enjoyable food can be!

At first this will require a little more thought than it did before. You'll have to be more creative in what you cook or order. You'll have to choose low-fat foods for yourself and leave the deep-dish pie for someone else. You'll have to be careful to feast until you're full, but not beyond.

But since you have been cutting out fat and sugar and excess from your diet all along, you will find you now need less to get the same pleasurable effect. Overindulgence will cease to hold the same appeal.

A good meal with friends is still one of the greatest blessings.

MARCH 27

Better is the enemy of good. —VOLTAIRE

Perfection is a moving target that ultimately becomes a trap for those who pursue it. When you have done a good job, take real pleasure in it. Don't be stingy in giving praise just because you could have done a little better, perhaps swimming two more laps at the pool or stopping with one bite less of food. You did just fine. You don't want to be the parent who overlooks the five A's on her child's report card and punishes him for the one A-minus, do you?

Never being satisfied is a crime against myself.

MARCH 28

You may have to fight a battle more than once to win it. —MARGARET THATCHER

Have you been here before? Have you had the experience of losing and gaining back the same ten pounds (or more)? If so, you may still be regarding this weight-reduction program with trepidation, wondering whether you can make your weight loss stick. You've disappointed yourself so many times already.

The answer to the question, "What makes this time different?" is "Everything." You've learned important lessons from the past (for example, that all the fasting and quick-weight-loss diets in the world won't help you maintain your ideal weight permanently), and you're applying that knowledge now. No matter how many times you have "failed" before, all it takes to succeed now is one more attempt.

*I have learned from my past experiences, an?
that knowledge will help me succeed this tir*

To dream of the person you would like to be is to waste the person you are. —ANONYMOUS

You have straight hair and you wish it were curly. You're enviably tall, but you'd give your long legs for a petite figure any day. No matter who we are, we can fall into the trap of wanting to be somebody else.

Try looking at what you have and seeing the beauty in it. What can you do to make it even better? Work with the grain of your being, rather than going against it. Appreciate the richness of what is already yours!

Everything I need I already have.

Vice goes a long way toward making life bearable. A little vice now and then is relished by the best of men. —FINLEY PETER DUNNE

A smidgen of something "bad" now and then can give you a thrill that's worth the price of admission. A little vice, now and then. Not a lot, a little. What a refreshing thought in this age of controls and limitations.

Stay away from the thing that's going to send you over the edge and into a downward spiral. Choose something to indulge in that's well within your ability to say no to when you've had enough. Maybe it's a trashy novel or an ice-cold, extra-dry martini. Whatever it is, make it something you'll really enjoy. Be creative!

Without feeling I need to wallow in it, I'll let myself be human and enjoy a little vice now and then.

Guard your heart more than any treasure, for it is the source of all life. —PROVERBS 4:23

Sometimes we ignore our better judgment and get involved with the wrong people when we know in advance this is a mistake. If we've already gotten the message, why go through the painful experience? We're taking ourselves through hard lessons that we really don't need.

It's not necessary to batter our hearts with emotional roller coasters and bumper-car rides. We can also treat ourselves gently and insist that others do the same.

I can save myself for those who will treat me well in return.

APRIL 1

Creative minds have always been known to survive any kind of bad training.

—ANNE FREUD

We are not, as we are often told, doomed to repeat our past.

We may have been abused by our parents. Or maybe their only serious flaw was that they instilled in us a love of white-trash cooking. But whatever our upbringing, we have survived it thus far. And we can rise above it, too.

If a behavior that we learned as a child no longer works for us, we can alter it. We are creative beings, and as such are highly adaptable to new experiences and surroundings. Each day we make a choice in how we live.

I may not have been given everything I needed as a child, but I have the ability to seek it out now.

Learn what you are, and be such. —PINDAR

An ancient Greek myth tells of the powerful warrior Achilles, who was invulnerable to his enemies everywhere except on the heel of his foot. We each have our Achilles' heel—some area of vulnerability that can bring us down even in the face of great resolve. What is your Achilles' heel? Are you tempted to overeat while experiencing emotions such as anxiety or boredom, or during activities such as watching TV?

We may not be able to eliminate our weaknesses. Consequently, we must learn to live with them and protect ourselves from them, especially when we find ourselves in situations where we are vulnerable to eating binges. One practical way to do this is to eat regular, satisfying meals that keep hunger under control in the first place. We can also keep nonfat snack foods around the house for those times when self-control falls by the wayside.

Some bad habits can't be changed, but I can learn to manage them.

The uneasiness of hunger can be more quickly removed by a bowl of good soup than by any other variety of food. —J. B. AND L. E. LYMAN

Soup as a first course, soup as the main dish. When you want to take the edge off a ravenous appetite, soup is the food of choice. Eat up!

As long as you stay away from those with cream-based broths and fatty meats as ingredients, soups are healthful and low in calories and fat. You can easily make your own with canned broth, some chopped vegetables, and condiments of your choice. Tailor soups to the season: root vegetables in winter, early harvest crops in spring, and the full selection of vegetables and fruits available in summer and fall.

Soup is also a good food to order in restaurants as an appetizer. By the time you get to the main course, you'll already be feeling full.

When I'm feeling as though I might overeat, I'll help myself to a cup of broth or bowl of soup to ward off hunger.

The sin of perfectionism is that it mutilates life by demanding the impossible.
—JEROME FRANK

When you watch the Olympic Games, you see athletes at the top of their form. They give outstanding—sometimes even inspired—performances. They reach for perfection. Rarely, if ever, however, do they attain it.

Even the finest gold-medal performance includes a misstep or a turn that was a bit too wide. What looks like perfection is an illusion—just ask the athlete, who will remember everything that went wrong.

Will they enjoy their successes, or rather let their mistakes haunt them? The same question applies to you. Reaching perfection is impossible. Instead, work to the best of your ability under the conditions you face at the time. Look at your mistakes and learn from them—but don't punish yourself for them. Mistakes are an inevitable part of taking chances.

Perfection is relative and remains ever out of reach. Instead, I strive to do my best.

Live so that you can stick out your tongue at the insurance doctor. —DON MARQUIS

To some extent, our health is determined by what we feed our bodies and how we take care of our other needs. Yes, there are illnesses and accidents that are out of our control, but those who have built up their strength through healthy living are less likely to be felled—or even attacked —by disease.

What is healthy living? Moderation in your eating and drinking, adequate sleep, and regular exercise. Less tangible but just as important are things like a job that suits you, friends and family with whom you share love, and outside activities that give you pleasure.

Your reward for healthy living is increased vitality and less time at the doctor's office. And you'll have the satisfaction of knowing you did your part in making the good life happen.

I will live to maintain good health.

The art of selfishness consists in looking after your own needs so that no one else will have to. —DAVID SEABURY

In our society, calling someone selfish is considered an insult. Certainly someone who thinks *only* of herself is no great addition to the world. But there's a way of being selfish that's just the opposite of being a burden to others. You take care of your own needs, quietly, without ceremony. Now you are free to take care of others.

Only when our own needs are taken care of do we really have anything to share freely with others. The woman who feeds her family, but never sits down to enjoy the meal herself places a burden of guilt on those she loves. But when she takes care of herself she gives them the example of self-love.

I treat myself well so that I can have something to share with others.

Obesity is a mental state, a disease brought on by boredom and disappointment. The one way to get thin is to reestablish a purpose in life.
—CYRIL CONNOLLY

Boredom and disappointment are the nemeses of the dieter. Are you living with a real purpose, or has your life lost its meaning and satisfaction? What have you done for the betterment of your person today? For another? For society? How many hobbies and projects are you planning to start sometime in the future —and the future never seems to arrive?

It's so easy for those concerned about their weight to become food-obsessed. Food-obsessed people worry about whether they should eat something, and then feel guilty about having eaten it. They live from meal to meal: breakfast to coffee break to lunch to snack to dinner to dessert.

Are you eating to avoid living? Are you food-obsessed? If so, it's time to move your focus elsewhere.

Today I will take steps toward reaching a goal and finding my purpose in life.

A smiling face is half the meal.
— LATVIAN PROVERB

Does your family race through a meal, or perhaps not even dine together? Are family arguments and bickering typical dinner-table fare? Do you eat standing up in the kitchen or plunked down in front of the television? Or do you, at least a few times a week, share a good meal with others and use the time to connect with them and talk about the happenings of your day, your thoughts, and your feelings?

Food is a gift I share with others as often as I can.

A successful individual typically sets his next goal somewhat, but not too much, above his last achievement. In this way he steadily raises his level of aspiration. — KURT LEWIN

So you've lost a few pounds and inches? Congratulations. Now you can aim to lose a few more.

Perhaps it's getting a little easier now that you're in the groove. High-fat foods hold less appeal, and you look forward to exercise, rather than dread it. So should you accelerate your goals? Cut back even more on your consumption?

Whoops, not so fast. Tempting as it may be to rush things along at this point, you're still better off taking it easy. The time it takes to lose the weight is not time wasted if you use it to establish new and better habits.

Setting realistic goals will help me establish good habits for life.

In nature there are neither rewards nor punishments —there are consequences.
—ROBERT G. INGERSOLL

For many of us, eating is as much an emotional experience as a physical one. We eat to comfort ourselves, and then feel worse afterward for breaking a diet. We "reward" ourselves with ice cream one day, then "punish" ourselves for the indulgence with a diet of celery and carrot sticks the next. And then console ourselves for the deprivation with a bag of chips the day after. And on and on.

Try to defuse some of the emotion connected with food in your life. Overeating is a bad habit —not a crime. When you slip up, it doesn't help either to beat yourself up about it or go to extremes the next day.

Instead, every time you begin to put food in your mouth, remember: If I consume more than my body needs today, I will gain weight. If I eat to satisfy my physical hunger and no more, eventually I will reach my ideal weight. It's a law of nature —cause and effect. It's really as simple as that.

Starting today, I will resist the urge to punish or reward myself for my eating behavior. Learning to accept mistakes and move on is an important lesson for all areas of my life.

Man lives not by material bread alone.
—HINDUISM

It's easy to get so wrapped up in earning our daily bread that we forget to feed our souls. Sometimes we find ourselves alone in front of an open refrigerator late at night, trying to fill the void inside us with food. But our appetites seem to be insatiable, a bottomless pit. We need *soul* food, too, but starve ourselves spiritually by settling for a poor substitute.

When we realize that we are bingeing on food in an attempt to satisfy our spiritual hunger, the best thing we can do is stop. To eat until we are sick is pointless because the soul's hunger will never be satisfied by food for the body alone.

What can we do instead to take care of our spiritual needs? The answer is different for each person, but many find spiritual nourishment in prayer. Prayer can take many forms: a meditation, a chant, a kind act, a song, a shared church service.

If my hunger is spiritual, I will give nourishment to my soul, so I can truly be satisfied.

One loses so many laughs by not laughing at oneself. —SARA JEANNETTE DUNCAN

You're about to make a presentation to a new boss or meet a blind date. You're nervous and want everything to go perfectly. Everything is going along just fine, when suddenly you trip, and fall unceremoniously to the floor. How do you react?

If your answer is that you have a good laugh with the other person, get up, and put the blunder behind you—congratulations! By letting go of the tremendous burden of perfectionism, you've given yourself a refreshing lift. When you can laugh at the things about yourself that you usually take so seriously, you've admitted yourself back into the human race, where everyone makes mistakes, and all of us look silly now and then.

When I can laugh at my fears and worries, I lessen the power they hold over me.

Losing an illusion makes you wiser than finding a truth. —LUDWIG BORNE

We are so good at fooling ourselves. Those of us who are perfectionists believe that if we try hard enough, we really can get it all right. And that means being perfect. No mistakes allowed.

What a sham. We have never (for more than a moment, anyway) achieved perfection. Chances are we never will, for life is constantly in flux. The only perfection is in living in the moment.

We can begin to grow up only when we let go of our illusions of perfection and allow life to unfold as it will.

I have nothing to lose by letting go of my illusions. I never gained anything from them anyway.

APRIL 14

No one can make you feel inferior without your consent. —ELEANOR ROOSEVELT

Every time you find yourself saying "He made me feel that way," or "She's driving me crazy," stop yourself and listen to what you're saying.

By blaming other people for your reactions, you feel justified in them. But the truth is, outside events do not cause you to feel or act a certain way. You choose what you are going to do. If someone screams at you, for example, you have numerous options: You can scream back, respond calmly, walk away, go to the refrigerator, call a friend to talk to about it, write a letter, or go out for a run—whatever.

Learn to take charge of your own feelings. You have more control than you think.

I can control my responses to life's events.

APRIL 15

Fashion condemns us to many follies; the greatest is to make oneself its slave.
—NAPOLEON BONAPARTE

For women at least, thin is in right now. (In Bonaparte's time, a little more plumpness was considered a beauty ideal.) Small breasts, large breasts, tiny hips, skinny legs, shapely hourglass figures: At one time or another in the past four decades all have been in favor. Fashions change. They may or may not be in sync with your body's natural shape. So why let your feelings about your body be governed by arbitrary standards that other people devise?

I possess my own unique beauty.

APRIL 16

Be thine own palace, or the world's thy jail.
— JOHN DONNE

Get into the habit of treating yourself like a king or queen. Spend as much time taking care of your body as you do taking care of your other responsibilities. Pay attention to good grooming and regular physical conditioning. Allowing yourself pleasure in the physical realm is important when you're trying to cut down on eating and get your body in shape. Your incentive to lose weight grows as you improve your relationship with your body. When you feel good about yourself in your body you feel better about yourself in the world.

What would make me feel like a king or queen? Is it something I can do for myself each week?

APRIL 17

Sometimes the most urgent and vital thing you can possibly do is take a complete rest.
— ASHLEIGH BRILLIANT

We push ourselves so hard—and for what? Whom are we trying to please?

Taking care of your own health is just as important as taking care of everyone else's. When you're exhausted, it's time to stop the merry-go-round and get off for a few days of rest. You're no good to anyone else when your energy is depleted, and you're especially no good to yourself.

When you return well-rested, you will find to your amazement that all of your charges will in the meantime have learned to take care of themselves. Sure, they'll be glad to have you back. But now you will see more clearly what you need to do, and what you should allow others to do for themselves.

I owe it to myself and others to take care of myself.

The only way to get rid of a temptation is to yield to it. Resist it, and your soul grows sick with longing for the things it has forbidden to itself. —OSCAR WILDE

There are times when you can practice self-control successfully, and other times when damage control is all you can hope for. You will know those times when they arrive: The obsession for a particular food takes over your consciousness, and suddenly it's all you can think of. It's likely to be a food that's wildly inappropriate in a weight-loss program.

If you're in the throes of an irrational food craving that just won't go away, it may be best to give in before it gains too much power over you. Take it slowly. See if a bite or two is all you need. Stop at a small serving and walk away. Was that enough to satisfy? Keep asking yourself this question until the answer is yes, and then put the rest out of sight.

After the craving has subsided, don't make the mistake of throwing in the towel, even if you feel you've blown it big-time. Start again, now. In the bigger picture, this is just part of the process.

I will take back the power I have given to certain foods.

In America we eat, collectively, with a glum urge for food to fill us. We are ignorant of flavor. We are, as a nation, taste-blind.
—M. F. K. FISHER

Food writer M. F. K. Fisher spent her formative years fine-tuning her palate and culinary skills in France. Her many books describe a love affair with food that lasted a lifetime. She understood food intimately, and like other serious cooks, was able to create new dishes because she had trained herself to pay attention to flavors and how they interact.

Do you really taste the food you eat, or do you "eat with a glum urge for food to fill"? Are you cheating yourself out of a sensory experience by scarfing down your meals instead of mindfully paying attention to what you are taking in?

Is the food I consume truly good-tasting, or am I just eating to feel full?

Sanity is very rare; every man almost, and every woman, has a dash of madness.
—RALPH WALDO EMERSON

We all feel a little insane sometimes. Certain people or situations seem to bring this on. The trick is to get through it without resorting to destructive behaviors, such as abusing food or chemical substances. A first step is to accept madness as a legitimate part of our psyches. We don't have to snuff it out. We can listen to what it is telling us.

We can even appreciate our touch of insanity for the way it shakes up our thinking. How dull life would be without a little bit of craziness and turmoil! Isn't a dash of madness in us the salt that gives the dish of life its flavor?

Normal is a relative term. We all have our own quirks.

We judge ourselves by our motives and others by their actions. —DWIGHT MORROW

We're so hard on ourselves! We know all of our temptations and how many times we've come close to giving in to them. Often we enter those struggles in the "loss" column, even if we ultimately won the battle. We find it hard to separate the internal conflict from the end result, and so we do not give ourselves the credit we deserve.

Do we really think that other people act without internal struggles? They too have their close calls and their selfish moments. We just don't see them happening.

It's time to give credit where credit is due.

Anyone who overlooks the instincts will be ambuscaded by them. —CARL JUNG

Our bodies will very clearly tell us what we need if we will only listen to what they are saying. They respond with fear when we are in dangerous situations. They bristle up when we are being attacked. But we have learned to ignore the signals and now we are paying the price.

Retrain yourself to sense your body's reactions. Don't judge or suppress them if they don't make immediate sense. Just take note of how you feel and then, later on, watch how the situation develops. Was your body communicating useful information? What if you always paid attention to these impulses?

Instinct is my body's way of communicating complex information in a shorthand form.

Do not miss a day's enjoy or forgo your share of innocent pleasure. —ECCLESIASTICUS 14:14

What constitutes a weight-loss program? Good diet and exercise, of course. But there's another component that often gets overlooked: pleasure. Just as it is important to learn to eat well and get exercise, it is also important to learn how to take pleasure in your body—not necessarily the X-rated variety, just everyday, ordinary physical sensations. Treat yourself to pleasurable activities such as back rubs, scalp massages, and barefoot walks through tall grass. Pay regular attention to your body's well-being, and it will return the favor a hundredfold.

The third component of my weight-loss program is learning to take pleasure in my body.

All that I know, I learned after I was thirty.
—GEORGES CLEMENCEAU

What a relief to turn thirty! Yes, even in this culture of youth, where the face-lift and fashion industries seem to be conspiring to keep us twenty-two forever.

There's such power in finally reaching the point where you know a little more about who you are. You can stop pretending to be someone else—especially the someone advertising agencies want you to be. You can finally start to put away the "shoulds" and give yourself to what you truly want to do and be.

Beauty resides in those who know who they are and celebrate it.

APRIL 25

A good indignation brings out all one's powers.
—RALPH WALDO EMERSON

We swallow our pride, eat our words, and get fed up. This vivid imagery describes how we sometimes deal with our emotions: We take them in the gut.

But maybe all this emotional energy can be used toward more productive ends. Anger can be used to persuade others to change a situation we find infuriating. Fear gives us that edge to excel in new situations. Anxiety tips us off that maybe we're on the wrong track and need to rethink our position.

Even negative emotions can serve us well if we utilize their power.

APRIL 26

Success is getting what you want; happiness is wanting what you get. —DALE CARNEGIE

We live in a consumer society that is constantly stoking our desire for more, more, more. Is it any wonder we are often dissatisfied when we finally attain what it is we thought we wanted?

We can learn to be satisfied with who we are, and what we are, today. As soon as we let go of the myth that something we don't yet have (a new car? a promotion? weight loss?) is going to make us happy, we will, ironically, find ourselves happier than ever. For the first time, we will begin to appreciate the many subtle gifts we receive (in the past, they went unnoticed) each day.

What gifts can I be thankful for today?

There are as many nights as days, and the one is just as long as the other in the year's course. Even a happy life cannot be without a measure of darkness, and the word happy *would lose its meaning if it were not balanced by sadness.*
—CARL JUNG

We live in a society that worships happiness and treats sadness as if it were an aberration or a disease. But what a sensible perspective Jung offers here: Happiness and sadness are both normal parts of the cycle of life.

Keep his words in mind the next time you are feeling down. If you are sad, perhaps it is for a specific reason. Without the feeling of sadness, you would never know what was wrong. Best not to smother it with drink, drugs, or overeating. Pay attention to what it is telling you about your life. Then let the emotion drift away naturally, like the clouds over your head.

Sadness and happiness are intertwined; one cannot exist without the other.

Real joy comes not from ease or riches or from the praise of men, but from doing something worthwhile. —WILFRED T. GRENFELL

Sometimes the hunger we are trying to satisfy is not physical, but spiritual hunger that comes from a lack of meaning in our lives. So we keep eating and eating, but the hunger never goes away. Not until we find a greater purpose for our lives do we begin to satiate the gnawing feeling we have inside.

It's not enough just to earn a lot of money, or attain great celebrity in your field. All of us need to feel that what we do matters, makes a difference in the world somehow. The satisfaction often doesn't come from our careers but from our outside interests. For one person, it means devoting free time to painting watercolors, for another, it comes from working for environmental causes. What gives meaning to your life?

What special gift can I offer the world while I am here?

We sit at breakfast, we sit on the train on the way to work, we sit at work, we sit at lunch, we sit all afternoon . . . a hodgepodge of sagging livers, sinking gall bladders, drooping stomachs, compressed intestines, and squashed pelvic organs. —JOHN BUTTON, M.D.

We hardly need to move a muscle to get anywhere today. Cars, trains, buses, planes, escalators, and elevators all take us where we need to go. And once we get there, we probably won't be going anywhere fast: most of our jobs are sedentary, keeping us sitting at a desk eight hours or more each day.

Our bodies just weren't made for this inactivity; they need to move and stretch. Forget what magazine articles say about exercising three times a week —you need to get on your feet and walk, run, or stroll every day. Stretch your torso, relax your neck, take some deep breaths, and work up a light sweat. You don't need to finish a marathon. You just gotta get up outta that chair!

I will respect my body's need for movement.

Take a music-bath once or twice a week for a few seasons, and you will find that it is to the soul what the water-bath is to the body.
—OLIVER WENDELL HOLMES

What a beautiful image Holmes creates here. Picture the scene: You are reclining in a comfortable chair. Music is washing over you in waves, cleansing and refreshing your soul.

What type of music is playing? What does the room look like? Is it light or dark outside? What are you wearing? How do you feel?

Music has a powerful effect on our senses. Think of the difference between a nightclub and a church service and you can imagine what an important role music plays in creating a mood. We turn to it when we're jazzed or sad or sitting bored in traffic. Often it is just in the background. Try focusing on it sometime, when you have a few minutes to relax. Put on some music you enjoy, lie back, close your eyes, and let it take you away. See how good it makes you feel.

Music is a tonic for my soul.

May 1

We were taken to a fast-food cafe where our order was fed into a computer. Our hamburgers, made from the flesh of chemically impregnated cattle, had been broiled over counterfeit charcoal, placed between slices of artificially flavored cardboard, and served to us by recycled juvenile delinquents.

—JEAN-MICHEL CHAPEREAU

Through the strength of advertising and our own self-delusion, we have somehow come to believe that our fast-food meals taste good. Yet, if we were to look at these foods more carefully—study their origins and really savor their taste—we would find them less desirable, possibly even disgusting.

Think of Chapereau's description the next time you're tempted by the convenience or habit of a drive-through restaurant. Take a minute to think about the food you will be taking into your body—chemically flavored sugar water, fat- and salt-saturated potato puree, nearly flavorless meat that has been injected with hormones and who knows what else. Consider the lack of nutrients and the huge quantity of fat and calories you will be consuming.

And if you decide to eat it anyway, you will at least be conscious of your decision. Next time it may not taste so good.

I will think about what I am feeding my body before I put it into my mouth.

Friendship, like love, is the most important bread and butter for life. —ANGNA ENTERS

Friends sustain us when we're feeling down. They remind us of who we are. They share in our accomplishments and offer their hands to us when we trip and fall. They confide their dreams. They listen to our fears. They grow up with us and grow old with us. They watch over our children. They challenge us to do the right thing. They give love and do not expect perfection in return. They are imperfect themselves. They are what we sometimes are not able to be for ourselves.

Food is no substitute for good friends.

Even were a cook to cook a fly, he would keep the breast for himself. —POLISH PROVERB

Are you the woman who prepares dinner each night for your family, but never stops serving others long enough to sit down to eat yourself? Do you give yourself life's leftovers, while giving the best portions to anyone and everyone else before you? Wise up!

There's nothing honorable in neglecting yourself for other people. You're only communicating the message that you're not worth a whole lot to yourself. And if that's the case, your gift is not worth a whole lot either. But if you respect yourself enough to take care of yourself, your kindness to others will be cherished as the valuable gift that it is.

In my desire to serve, I will remember to take care of myself, too.

MAY 4

Hunger is not debatable. —HARRY HOPKINS

It's important, expecially while you are in the midst of weight loss, to get enough to eat. Not just for nutrition, though that is vital, but to make it as easy as possible for you to continue your program.

Skipping meals or starving yourself will only weaken your resolve. When your blood sugar dips low, and your hunger rises, all the resolutions in the world will not be effective in keeping you from reaching for the first edible thing that presents itself. And it could just as easily be a worthless candy bar as a bowl of nutritious beans.

I will keep myself properly fed with low- or nonfat foods to reduce my temptation to binge.

MAY 5

We have to learn to be our own best friends because we fall too easily into the trap of being our worst enemies. —RODERICK THORP

Some people use excess weight as an excuse to punish themselves. Do you feel bad when you overeat? Are you ready to start feeling good instead?

Observe your own actions today. Every time you eat or do something, ask yourself if it makes you feel good or bad about yourself. If you find that many things, including overeating, actually make you feel quite bad, it's time to make some changes. Approach each day mindfully, asking yourself, "What action would make me feel good about myself right now?" The path to feeling better about yourself will become quite clear.

I'm ready to start feeling good about myself.

MAY 6

The main thing is that you hear life's music everywhere. Most people hear only its dissonances. —THEODOR FONTANE

People sometimes laugh at the concept of using positive thinking to reach our goals. But to make headway in a new direction, we must have hope. We must have a reason to persist in our dreams. It's not a matter of whitewashing all that we see. It's enough that we keep our hearts open so that we can appreciate the full spectrum of what life contains. We need the ability to perceive its beauty and goodness, as well as all the things that can go wrong.

Some people listen for the wrong notes in life's music. I want to hear the whole song.

MAY 7

If it keeps up, man will atrophy all his limbs but the push-button finger.

—FRANK LLOYD WRIGHT

Laborsaving devices are doing us in! It's gotten to the point where we're riding elevators to get to the stair-stepping machines at the gym.

Why not rebel and take back your body? Search for a parking spot far from the supermarket entrance. Put away the remote and get up to change the channel on the TV instead. Walk instead of ride; use a hand tool where a power tool might do; lift, pull, and carry whenever possible.

Why get caught up in following the crowd off the cliff? Chart your own path —the longer one—and save yourself while you can.

I show love for my body by using it.

Every man is a consumer and ought to be a producer. —RALPH WALDO EMERSON

We've become so disconnected from our food sources. Our supermarket food is picked too early, processed, shot up with preservatives, shrink-wrapped. We've lost the sense of where it comes from and how it is grown.

You can develop a new appreciation for food by growing some of your own. Strawberries are even more tender and delicately sweet when you harvest them yourself. A dash of fresh herbs can be snipped fresh from your garden before each meal. You can watch your tomatoes ripen on the vine to full maturity.

When you grow your own food, you see that food is not just a product to be bought and blindly consumed. It is life sustaining our lives.

Food is most nutritious when it is eaten closest to its natural state.

I do not pray for a lighter load, but for a stronger back. —PHILLIPS BROOKS

Almost anything is possible if we believe it is so. We can build up the strength of our resolve by giving ourselves rewards for our successes along the way. A steady flow of positive feedback is to the dieter what a daily exercise program is to the backpacker about to embark on a long trip.

Give yourself encouragement for keeping up your program: a mental pat on the back at the end of the day, an inexpensive gift to yourself or a special outing you enjoy at the end of each week. Treat yourself to a spa weekend when you hit an important milestone. Reward yourself for the effort; don't hold out until you achieve perfect results.

I will give myself as much encouragement as I can. Positive, not negative, reinforcement is what will carry me through.

The need for beauty is as positive a natural impulse as the need for good. —LUTHER BURBANK

Let's not move so fast through life that we neglect to adorn our lives with the beautiful touches that bring so much pleasure to us and to those around us.

Bring fresh flowers into the house. Put art on your walls. If you enjoy sewing, spend a few hours making special curtains for your child's room. Tailor your office or den so that it is a comfortable and pleasing place in which to read or work on your computer. Keep your front yard in good order so you communicate a positive message to your neighbors, too.

There is goodness in beauty. I will make room for it in my life.

Live as if everything you do will eventually be known. —HUGH PRATHER

Now this is a scary one, particularly for those accustomed to hoarding secret meals. But it certainly is a good practice. And not only in the sense that we must be accountable for our "sins."

The habit of concealing our private self from others reflects a schism in our lives. We show that we value our relationship with food over our relationships with other people when we conceal the real facts about our eating habits. We feel alienated from others when we hide our truths, even from those closest to us.

In protecting myself from the disapproval of others, I also lose the opportunity to receive their support.

Strange how one's thoughts turn to food when there is nothing else to think of.
—John Colton and Clemence Randolph

When was the last time you took a class on a subject you wanted to learn more about? Turned off the TV sitcom and picked up a good book instead? Spent a Sunday with your kids at the science museum?

If you're not doing enough to feed your mind, chances are you often find yourself bored. It's in this state that food obsessions thrive.

The next time you find yourself thinking about a frozen cheesecake, try this instead. Take out a piece of paper and a pencil. Write down three things you've always wanted to do or to learn about. Skip the cheesecake and try initiating one of those activities instead.

When you finish, you may still crave the cheesecake—but maybe not. Or perhaps you'll be satisfied with just a small portion.

I will combat boredom by stimulating my mind and opening myself up to new learning opportunities.

Happiness in this world, when it comes, comes incidentally. Make it the object of pursuit, and it leads us on a wild-goose chase, and is never attained. Follow some other object, and very possibly we may find that we have caught happiness without dreaming of it.

—NATHANIEL HAWTHORNE

How can you capture anything as ethereal as happiness and expect it to stay? The answer is, you can't. It comes, it goes, it haunts us in its absence, it circles around us in our memories. It visits us when we least expect it. It's not something we can depend on, but when we remove our expectations of attaining it, we can enjoy it when it comes our way.

Happiness is something I can't control, and that is part of its charm.

Make it a rule never to come to the table in a churlish mood. —SOLON ROBINSON

It's a bad idea to eat when you're feeling angry or frustrated. You'll wolf down your food and won't even taste it. Your digestion will be poor because of all your churning emotions. If you're eating with others, you'll ruin their meal, too.

Instead, take a fifteen-minute walk to ease through some of the excess emotions, or spend a few minutes in deep breathing and meditation. Talk with someone who will listen patiently and let you blow off steam. You're ready to eat when you've calmed down.

I will make it a practice not to swallow my anger or lash out at others during a meal.

Tomorrow is often the busiest day of the week.
—SPANISH PROVERB

We all know this one, don't we? "I blew it today, but I'll start my diet over again . . . tomorrow." That means that today we'll be loading up on all those forbidden foods we've sworn we won't eat in the future. We consume twice as much as we need in anticipation of starving ourselves tomorrow—one day of pull-out-the-stops feasting, followed by weeks of fasting and atonement.

Most of us already know this approach doesn't really work. Tomorrow we will feel guilty for overeating today, or resentful of the bad deal we've cut for ourselves. (One day of feasting for a lifetime of deprivation? What a terrible fate!) Soon we'll find ourselves raiding the refrigerator to soothe our anxious nerves.

This is erroneous thinking. Something in us still believes that an overindulgence in food holds emotional rewards. As long as we rely on food to manage our emotions, we will be caught in the endless cycle of starve and binge.

It's time to break the cycle. I will practice moderation in my eating today and tomorrow.

A good meal ought to begin with hunger.
—FRENCH PROVERB

Some compulsive eaters never experience hunger at all, but nibble at this and that throughout the day. More than a few are propelled by anxiety, boredom, or fear into eating when they're not hungry—using food as a balm or a comfort. Some are in the habit of breakfast at eight, lunch at noon, and dinner at six—whether they're hungry or not. Others blame the business lunches, cocktail parties, and family celebrations they have to attend, where the temptations to overeat are many.

But if you watch those who are at their ideal weight, you'll notice a pattern. They don't eat unless they are hungry. Sure, you may catch them at a company party sampling all the hors d'oeuvres. Sometimes you'll see them piling their plates high at the buffet or salad bar. But as many times as not, they're also the ones who say no to the box of chocolates circulating the office during the holidays. While everyone else at a cocktail party is eating greasy chicken wings and peanuts, they'll content themselves with a glass of mineral water. They eat when they're hungry and they don't when they're not.

I will enjoy food more when hunger is my companion at the meal.

Good breathing is of utmost value in maintaining good body tone. —GENE TUNNEY

When you're feeling tired, stressed, or scattered, take a few moments to do some yoga breathing. Slowly draw air in through your nose, filling your lungs so deeply your abdomen actually expands. Hold the breath a few counts, and then just as slowly let it go, pushing it out completely, through your mouth. Repeat the process.

You will increase the oxygen flow to every muscle, cell, and organ in your body. Your mind will feel clearer, your energy will rise, your mood will lift.

Breath is life: I will work toward improving my breathing throughout the day.

Half a man's life is devoted to what he calls improvements, yet the original had some quality which is lost in the process. —E. B. WHITE

In our longing for change, we may be tempted to throw away everything we were before and start from scratch. But when we make such a radical move, not only do we risk losing our bearings, we may undervalue some wonderful traits we have always possessed. Most of what we have been in the past is worth hanging onto. We don't have to lose those good qualities when we lose weight. Just as we can let go of the things that no longer work for us, we can take whatever we want into our new lives as well.

The fact that I have come this far shows strength of character. What other good traits do I possess?

MAY 19

The physically fit can enjoy their vices.
—LLOYD PERCIVAL

One of the wonderful things about exercise is that it allows us a greater margin for error in what we eat. When you get several good aerobic workouts each week, you can afford to eat a little more than if you were just sitting around. Not only are you burning off calories and fat while you exercise, but you're speeding up your resting metabolism for the whole day. So take every opportunity for moderate exercise that you can. You'll feel you've earned the privilege, when you indulge your vices now and then.

I am doing myself a favor by engaging in moderate exercise on a regular basis.

MAY 20

He that would have fruit must climb the tree.
—THOMAS FULLER

In the end, it all comes down to just doing the work. There's no getting around it. You have to be willing to say no to the gooey-rich chocolate chip cookies and yes to a moderate amount of exercise every day.

But the rewards for your work are there for you too. You can look forward to the beautiful clothes you'll be able to wear proudly and the energy you will feel as you get into better shape.

The rewards are waiting for me as I work toward my goal.

MAY 21

Is not sight a jewel? Is not hearing a treasure? Is not speech a glory? O my Lord, pardon my ingratitude and pity my dullness who am not sensible of these gifts. —THOMAS TRAHERNE

Give your taste buds a rest today and rediscover your senses of smell, sight, sound, and touch. Visit a rose garden in bloom; breathe in the intoxicating fragrance and look at the beauty of each flower. Take a walk through a park or a nature preserve. Set aside a few hours for a sport you enjoy. Afterward, relax in a sauna or whirlpool or hot bath. Treat yourself to a therapeutic massage.

Participate in a church service or other inspirational gathering where the music, words, and spirit will uplift you. Take time at the end of the day to relax and ponder. Give your children a hug tonight and read them bedtime stories; you'll all benefit from the closeness. Rekindle your relationship with your spouse or companion by getting away for a weekend by yourselves.

What riches are available to me in this miracle called life.

There is luxury in self-reproach. When we blame ourselves, we feel no one else has a right to blame us. —OSCAR WILDE

We think we have it figured out. If we're really hard on ourselves, we're safe from other people's judgments. If we dump on ourselves, no one else is going to. If we hurt ourselves, no one else can hurt us more.

Unfortunately, it doesn't work this way. What other people see is someone who's an open target for their abuse. They'll pile it on too. And even if they don't, they're not going to be impressed. It's no fun being around people who are always putting themselves down.

Stop beating yourself up. If you don't believe in yourself, who will?

I will resist the temptation to play the martyr and put myself down.

Simplify. —HENRY DAVID THOREAU

It's the litany of the 1990s: My life is so complicated. I don't have any time! All this rushing around can have negative implications for the person trying to lose weight. You rush through meals, grab whatever you can on the run. And when things get too hectic or stressful, you're vulnerable to overeating.

Thoreau had a good idea. If you often feel harried, why not look at your own life to see where you can cut back or get extra help? Activities you think are necessary may really be optional. Some things you do yourself could be delegated to others.

What is essential in my life, and what is just there taking up time?

We are more interested in making others believe we are happy than in trying to be happy ourselves. —FRANÇOIS LA ROCHEFOUCAULD

We care so much about what other people think of us. We work hard at proving to them that our lives are filled with great times, fun events, and snappy, happy people. We act as though we're in a television commercial for the good life.

Inside, we long for something that is authentic, a way of relating that is more honest. Our fear of vulnerability keeps us hiding behind a mask, but it is only when we are willing to take our masks off and admit who we really are that we have a chance of getting what we need.

I will stop trying to live my life to please other people. Instead, I will do what I need to do to please myself.

There are few hours in life more agreeable than the hour dedicated to the ceremony known as afternoon tea. —HENRY JAMES

Even while losing weight you can still enjoy the pleasures of a civilized meal with company. For the British, afternoon tea is a meal that's important to the leisure routine. For you, it may be Sunday brunch or supper. Don't cut this event out completely. But do take care of your diet needs while you observe it.

If high-fat foods usually dominate the menu, arrange for some special low- or nonfat foods you can enjoy. Keep the foods you want to avoid out of reach, so you won't be tempted. Realize that a big part of your enjoyment of these events is the conversation and ambiance. So look up from the food for awhile, and take time to appreciate these elements of the meal.

I will allow myself the pleasure of meals that have always been a part of my routine.

Success is to be measured not so much by the position that one has reached in life as by the obstacles which he has overcome while trying to succeed. —BOOKER T. WASHINGTON

In our goal-oriented society, we often believe that we have succeeded only when we have crossed the finish line. But when we look to the goal for our satisfaction we are likely to find ourselves disappointed. Real satisfaction comes with every battle won and every obstacle overcome.

Perverse as it may sound, try to enjoy the process of your weight loss. Reaching your goal weight is the culmination of many small successes along the way.

I take pleasure in each victory I achieve on the way to my goal.

You can take no credit for beauty at sixteen. But if you are beautiful at sixty, it will be your soul's own doing. —MARIE STOPES

Go to a mirror and look at your face: What do you see? Laugh lines or a scowl? A jaw set in bitterness or eyes sparkling with life?

Life deals its hand, and we respond gracefully, or we duke it out all the way. With each choice we make, we create our faces and we feed or starve our souls.

We recognize those truly beautiful people whose spirits shine through. We also know those who have atrophied inside and seem to have lost touch with their souls. Which one of these is you?

I will cultivate grace and beauty in my life.

He that has a great nose thinks everybody is speaking of it. —THOMAS FULLER

People who are overweight are typically hypersensitive about what other people think of them. If they wear something a little different or revealing, they imagine everyone staring at them and passing judgment. If a group walking behind them starts laughing, they immediately wonder if they are the source of the amusement. They feel that anyone looking in their direction is thinking negative things about them.

If you find yourself feeling this way, it's good to get a reality check. Strike up a conversation with the people you perceive as being hostile. Did they notice your outfit, or were they more concerned with what other people thought of *them*? Was that group laughing at you or at a private joke? Was the person gazing at you actually thinking that you looked like someone he'd like to get to know?

It's time to turn the spotlight off myself and put things in proper perspective.

No man is lonely while eating spaghetti—it requires so much attention.

—CHRISTOPHER MORLEY

So often we race through a meal, practically inhaling the food. By the time we've finished, we're ready for more because we didn't really taste what we just consumed.

Make each meal an active experience. Choose foods that involve all of your senses: crusty French bread that you tear off the loaf, steamy broths, spicy foods that clear your sinuses and give a kick going down. Arrange your food beautifully on the plate. Enjoy the scent of fresh herbs sprinkled on your food as a garnish. End your meal with a scoop of icy sherbet or sorbet.

Most important, take the time to enjoy your meal. Sit down to eat, always. Set a beautiful table, even for one. Improve your digestion by chewing your food thoroughly before swallowing. Taste what you put in your mouth.

Attention to the moment is a good habit to cultivate. By taking the time to concentrate on what I am eating, I will eat less and enjoy the meal more.

It seems to me that our three basic needs, for food and security and love, are so mixed and mingled and entwined that we cannot straightly think of one without the others. —M. F. K. FISHER

Some of us were raised in households where parents used food as a reward or a punishment. Others grew up in poor families where necessities—including food—were in short supply. Still others come from homes where food was plentiful, but love was scarce.

We are often unconscious of the relationship between food, love, and security in our lives. We are not aware that when we stuff ourselves with comfort foods, we may be trying to fill the emptiness in our gut that comes when love or security is missing. Unraveling the tangled braid of physical and emotional needs is an important step to gaining control of our overeating.

The next time I am tempted to eat when I am not physically hungry I will pay attention to what other need I may be trying to satisfy.

All changes, even the most longed for, have their melancholy, for what we leave behind us is a part of ourselves. We must die to one life before we can enter another. —ANATOLE FRANCE

Whether you believe it or not, fat has been your friend. It has given you protection in hostile environments where you felt unable to cope on your own. Food has provided comfort when no other could be found.

But now you are ready to change. You're facing life without the crutch of overeating. Acknowledge the significance of the change in your life. Feel grateful for the help overeating has given you, which you now no longer need. Accept the part of you that once did. And when you're ready, let it go.

Life is a process of constant change. I accept my past as part of my journey, even as I look ahead.

JUNE 1

Life's greatest happiness is to be convinced we are loved.
—VICTOR HUGO

Love is what all of us are seeking, isn't it? But often we search for it in roundabout ways. We work ourselves to death hoping for recognition, only to find that other people aren't all that impressed. We become masters of "nice," but that doesn't win people over either. We pretend we don't need anyone, but secretly hope someone will break through our defenses.

When you want to be loved, give love. Give it to yourself, your neighbor, your daughter, your ex-husband, your best friend. Give it freely, without expectations, obligations, or strings attached. It may not be returned to you in the way you had expected, but it will, definitely, come back.

It is in giving love that I receive love.

JUNE 2

Natural emotions can never be denied—only disguised.
— JOHN COLTON AND CLEMENCE RANDOLPH

If every extra pound on your body were an emotion you tried to suppress, what would your body be telling you right now? Would there be stories of the rage you were unable to express? The grief you never worked through? Your frustration with a situation you felt powerless to change?

When we experience an emotion, its energy cannot be denied. If we refuse to acknowledge a feeling, it only pops up somewhere else in disguise. When we're good at stuffing down our feelings with food, they show up as excess weight on our bodies.

I can enlist my body to help unlock my feelings.

JUNE 3

Clothes and manner do not make the man; but, when he is made, they greatly improve his appearance. — HENRY WARD BEECHER

As you slim down and move closer to your ideal weight, you will want to re-think the way you present yourself to the world. Experiment a little and see what works for you. Treat yourself to a new outfit, something you've never dared to wear before. Ask for a beauty makeover for your birthday and try out a new look. Spend a little more time grooming yourself, keeping your hair well-trimmed, your nails done, your clothes cleaned and pressed. Cultivate a pride in your appearance that may have been lacking when you felt ashamed of your weight.

My pride in myself shows in how I groom my body.

JUNE 4

It is something to be able to paint a particular picture, or to carve a statue, and so to make a few objects beautiful; but it is far more glorious to carve and paint the very atmosphere and medium through which we look. To affect the quality of the day—that is the highest of arts.
—HENRY DAVID THOREAU

Who says art has to be confined to a canvas or a pedestal? Take it to a bigger scale and treat your entire life as a work of art.

Put some real effort into living well: Not just cooking a meal, but preparing it artfully. Take care in decorating your home, landscaping your yard. Keep fresh flowers on your office desk. Wear clothes and jewelry that are uniquely you, perfumes and lotions that make you feel good. Put thought into the gifts you choose for your friends.

My life is a work of art that can be added to each day.

JUNE 5

When nobody around you seems to measure up, it's time to check your yardstick.
—BILL LEMLEY

When we judge everyone, including ourselves, by impossible standards, we set the stage for failure and disappointment. We never let anyone succeed, so what is the use of their trying? No one wants to put up with the abuse, so eventually they give up. We end up having do everything ourselves. Is that what we want?

It's great to have ideals, but unrealistic to think everyone shares them. Put a little slack into the expectations you have for others. And while you're at it, go a little easier on yourself as well.

Am I imposing overly high expectations on myself and other people?

Loneliness is and always has been the central and inevitable experience of every man.
—THOMAS WOLFE

There is no escaping loneliness. All of us feel it at one time or another. We are born and die alone, and throughout life face the fact of our aloneness repeatedly. Some Eastern religions believe that loneliness is just an illusion. They say we are really part of a singular consciousness in which all life is interconnected. Perhaps this is a bit abstract to be much consolation when we're sitting at home at night listening to the hum of the refrigerator. But maybe the thought that we are all in this together, all united by the fact of our aloneness, can give us some measure of comfort on those cheerless nights.

I am not alone in feeling lonely.

A life spent making mistakes is not only more honorable, but more useful than a life spent doing nothing. —GEORGE BERNARD SHAW

Critics sling their barbs from a safe, comfortable vantage point at the people who are out there taking chances. Yet the ones risking the ridicule are the people who come up with the new inventions, create the works of art, and solve the scientific puzzles. Be one of the brave ones. Go out on a limb. Do the thing you've never dared to do before. Play the fool, if you must. Make your time on earth mean something by investing yourself in it.

Who cares what other people think? In the end, you're the one who has to answer for your life. Better to look back on a life where much was attempted, rather than wondering in vain what your life would have been like if you'd only tried.

I will dive into experience and take my chances.

About a third of my cases are suffering from no clinically definable neurosis, but from the senselessness and emptiness of their lives.
—CARL JUNG

Therapy can be useful or even vital for working out some problems. It can help heal wounds, treat psychoses, and clarify values, among other things. One thing it can't do is create meaning in our lives. We have to do that ourselves. But how?

Helping other people is one way. Physicians now believe that doing a good turn for others even offers significant health benefits. It can be as casual or as formal as you like. Perhaps you can spend a little extra time listening when your troubled nephew has something on his mind. Or you can block out an afternoon each week to spend with an elderly person confined to bed. Or you can donate time to help poor residents establish a new community center. It's a truism, but when you give of yourself in this way, you will probably find you get back as much as you give.

How can I help others on a regular basis? What are the special skills and qualities that I have to offer?

When envy, hate, and fear are habitual, they are capable of starting genuine diseases.
— DR. ALEXIS CARREL

We've all seen the older person whose face seems locked in a perpetual scowl after years of foul moods. Well, just as our dispositions carve impressions on our faces, they also have an effect on our internal organs, some scientists believe.

When we experience negative emotions such as anger or fear, our immune system releases natural killer cells into our bloodstream to help us battle the enemy. Our heart is programmed to pump more blood, to enable us to run away or fight. These are normal processes. But when we keep our bodies in this state of stress for extended periods, physicians say, we wear out our organs and defense systems and we make ourselves more vulnerable to disease.

I will experience negative emotions as they arise and just as easily let them go.

When we do the best that we can, we never know what miracle is wrought in our life, or in the life of another. — HELEN KELLER

Have you ever run into a friend and found they had lost a lot of weight since you last saw them? What did you feel upon seeing them looking so great? Envious, perhaps? Maybe hopeful, as well: If Jill could take off the weight, so can I.

We never know how much our lives affect other people. As you lose weight and get in better shape, people will notice. Some will feel jealous, others will take pleasure in your accomplishment. Family members may feel relief that your health has improved. And you may also give other people hope, not just that they can lose weight, but that it is possible for all of us to change our lives for the better.

By helping myself I may be helping other people as well.

JUNE 11

Normal day, let me be aware of the treasure you are. Let me not pass you by in quest of some rare and perfect tomorrow. One day I shall dig my nails into the earth, or bury my face in the pillow, or stretch myself taut, or raise my hands to the sky, and want, more than all the world, your return. —MARY JEAN IRION

We will look back at these days, whose passing sometimes seems so painful, as our most valuable and fragile possession. Let us not wait until we encounter death to be grateful for the value of a life that hurries so quickly by.

When we live in the can't-wait-for-Friday mode, we are in essence wishing our lives away. No choice, you say? Not true. Everything you do is a choice. Your job is a choice. Your family is a choice. Your attitude is a choice. What would you choose on your deathbed if you could do it all again?

Each day is the most valuable thing I possess.

JUNE 12

I cannot give you the formula for success, but I can give you the formula for failure, which is—try to please everybody.

—HERBERT BAYARD SWOPE

Practice saying no today. Does it come easily? Or do you naturally want to keep the peace by agreeing to everything others want from you?

It's time to set limits—your own. Don't be so eager to say yes. When someone makes a request of you, say you need to think it over before you respond. Ask yourself if you have the time for this project. Do you have an interest in it? What does it offer you? Is the compensation adequate? Is this better suited for someone else?

Time is a finite resource to cherish and protect. The more time you spend engaged in activities you don't care about, the less time you have for those things you do.

I will please myself, then do what I can for other people.

Nothing in the world can take the place of persistence. —CALVIN COOLIDGE

The difference between those who are ultimately successful and those who aren't can be defined in just one word: persistence. Overnight success—that mythical experience—is so rare as to be almost nonexistent. What most of us don't see are the months or years of tough living, mundane jobs, and bad treatment that were endured before.

Often it is not the most talented who make it, it is the ones who can keep going through the hard times. The same thing holds true for weight loss. This is a marathon, not a fifty-yard dash. Pace yourself accordingly.

I will keep going, even when the going gets rough.

If one only wished to be happy, this could be easily accomplished; but we wish to be happier than other people, and this is always difficult, for we believe others to be happier than they are.
—MONTESQUIEU

We have a tendency to look at other people's lives as ideal and ours as lacking. You'd think we would learn, but we never seem to. We're always shocked when a scandal tears the lid off what seemed to be a "perfect" family and we get a peek inside to find it was anything but.

This is one of the dangers of comparing ourselves to others. We often measure ourselves against an unrealistic standard that even our idols never reach. This makes us feel ashamed of ourselves, disappointed. If only we could learn to be happy with what we have and stop searching outside ourselves for validation.

By comparing myself to other people I do no justice to myself.

JUNE 15

A man too busy to take care of his health is like a mechanic too busy to take care of his tools.
—SPANISH PROVERB

When we're young we can usually take our health for granted, and we often do. It's only when we start to lose our good health that we begin to appreciate its value.

Don't wait until your body is broken down before you pay attention to it. Keep it in good condition. Get enough sleep, eat nourishing foods, get regular exercise, and don't take yourself too seriously. Be the mechanic who cleans her tools and puts them away carefully every night after work, not the one who leaves them outside to be stolen or to rust in the cool night air.

I am never too busy to take care of my health.

JUNE 16

The superior man deliberates upon how he may walk in truth, not upon what he may eat.
—CONFUCIUS

Sometimes you will feel that your obsession with eating and overeating is just so much trivia, a self-indulgent concern that isn't worth the energy you put into it. And you're right.

As important as this issue is in life, it is only part of what we are. Yes, we need food to survive, and it's also a source of pleasure. But life is more than getting by and feeling good. Our lives are empty without attention to the spiritual realm.

The less I am concerned about food, the more time I have for more meaningful pursuits.

How do you accept your body—especially if you've been at war with it for years? Walk the walk of the Beautiful People. Buy the fashionable clothes. Wear the forbidden bathing suit. Go to the class reunion that's coming up. Make the appointment for the interview. Give the speech. Invite him over for a candlelight dinner. Accept the dates. Dance. Sing!

> —STEVEN C. STRAUSS, M.D., AND
> GAIL NORTH

If you are like many people who are—or who perceive themselves to be—overweight, these are things you just don't allow yourself. You worry that everyone will stare at your "enormous" thighs if you wear that bathing suit, so you cover up instead. Or you don't go out at all. Maybe you treat these events as rewards you'll give yourself when you've been "good" and lost the extra pounds.

Here's the rub: If you don't accept your body now, you are *not* going to accept it after you lose the weight. Once you reach your ideal weight, you'll still see a bulge here or a roll there that makes you self-conscious. You'll still be comparing your body to a magazine model's or your boyfriend's ideal or every woman you pass on the street. You'll be caught in the sliding scale of perfection. The closer you get, the further it moves out of reach.

Give yourself unconditional love *now*, as you are. Forget what people might be saying behind your back. Start doing those things you've always wanted to do. It's your life—why let somebody else set your limits?

Today I will stop living as a fat person and start living as the beautiful person that I am.

One remains young as long as one can still learn, can still take on new habits, can bear contradiction.

—MARIE VON EBNER-ESCHENBACH

We've all known them, the people who personify "old and crabby." Anything new is a threat, any interruption to their plans, a disturbance. New ideas? They haven't changed their opinions or tastes since their youth. Taking up a new interest or hobby is out of the question. They're stuck in a rut.

Don't be one of those people programmed to think of themselves as a finished work at age thirty or forty. No matter what your age, you are young as long as your mind and heart remain open. The next time you say to yourself, "I'm too old to change," reject the thought out of hand. What do you have to lose?

I will stay open to new attitudes about eating and exercise.

I am life that wants to live, in the midst of life that wants to live. —ALBERT SCHWEITZER

Those of us who live in cities or suburbs often feel ourselves disconnected from the rest of nature. We see ourselves as apart from nature, rather than as part of it.

Yet we possess the same life force that takes everything on earth through its cycle of living and dying. Plants rise from the soil in the spring. Birds are born and learn to fly. The ocean returns to the shore with each lapping wave. Our hearts beat, our lungs draw breath, our muscles contract and expand throughout the day.

Worries and anxieties may occupy our conscious minds, but life continues anyway. Our bodies know instinctively what to do. We are life that is part of a larger life.

I will step out of the way and let my instincts guide me.

Happiness belongs to those who are sufficient unto themselves. For all external sources of happiness and pleasure are, by their very nature, highly uncertain, precarious, ephemeral, and subject to chance. —ARTHUR SCHOPENHAUER

"I will be happy when I . . ." You've probably started a sentence like this before. What is the thing that you've vowed will make you happy? Getting out of debt? Finding a new job? Having a child? Losing forty pounds?

Achieving an external dream or goal will probably give you a great deal of satisfaction, but, ultimately, happiness will still be elusive. There will always be something else out there that you think you need.

As long as you look for happiness outside yourself it will remain out of reach. The need comes from inside and will be satisfied only by seeking its fulfillment there.

The only true happiness lies inside myself.

We suffer a lack of faith in ourselves that stems from judgment about our choices and failures of the past. —TOM RUSK, M.D.

You've failed yourself . . . over and over again. But you also have done good. Are you giving yourself credit for those times, or are you just focusing on what you don't like about yourself? It's so easy to overlook our accomplishments, large and small.

Try an experiment. Today, take note of every time you do something well, every time you make a good decision or resist a needless temptation. Write these things down if you can. At the end of the day, look over your list. Do you still feel you make mostly bad choices? Or does your version of reality need an adjustment?

Today and every day I will pay attention to the good things I do and the battles I win.

Success and failure are equally disastrous.
—TENNESSEE WILLIAMS

You've just been given the promotion you've sought for months. The party you gave over the weekend was a success. You stepped on the scale this morning to find that you've finally shed that stubborn ten pounds.

All happy events, right? So why do you feel so uneasy?

Success can be just as stressful as failure. Both bring change to our lives. When we make it to the top of the heap, part of us always knows we can just as easily fall off. What if I can't handle that job and am fired? Did I offend one of my guests with that comment I made as she was leaving? What if I slip up and gain back the ten pounds and more?

All of us have worries like this, and success—especially if we've never been comfortable with it before—can make them more pronounced. So if you feel uneasy, don't berate yourself for not being happy or content. Give yourself a little room to adjust to the changes in your life.

Anxiety about success is normal. I don't have to drown in my fears, but I will accept they are there.

JUNE 23

A big man is always accused of gluttony, whereas a wizened or osseous man can eat like a refugee at every meal, and no one ever notices his greed. —ROBERTSON DAVIES

When you're heavy and you eat with others, your extra weight is an uninvited guest at the table. You hesitate to eat with enjoyment, wondering what other people will think. Perhaps your parents used the dinner table as a soapbox to comment on your weight and eating habits. Now that you're an adult, people continue to comment or let their eyes speak for them.

It just isn't fair. You feel as though you have to answer for everything you put in your mouth, while your slender companion will not get a second glance chowing down a thick steak and fries.

Difficult as it is, you need to detach yourself from other people's judgments. Listen to your internal signals. Are you hungry or full? What does your body need right now? Let your body speak to you. Tune out the outside chatter.

My body knows best what it needs. Other people do not.

Every normal man must be tempted at times to spit on his hands, hoist the black flag, and begin slitting throats. —H. L. MENCKEN

Everyone experiences anger at some point, some more frequently than others. We may fantasize about "getting back" at the person with mean words, a harsh action, or even with violence. Other times we're just in a dark mood and want to take it out on someone. We may even be angry at ourselves and not know it.

Yet many of us were taught that anger is an inappropriate emotion. We don't have tools to deal with it, so we stuff it down, afraid of what we would do if we expressed it. Or we feel guilty when we get mad, thinking we have to be "nice" all the time.

When you feel angry, don't suppress it with food or drink or a fake smile. Instead, acknowledge the anger to yourself and see how it feels. Then take ten deep breaths to calm yourself. Ask yourself, "Should I express this now, or take a little time to cool off?" It often helps to write down how you feel. When the heat of the moment has passed, you will be ready to lower the black flag and deal with the situation in a more productive way.

Anger is a real emotion that needs to be acknowledged and accepted.

The people to whom we are support are those who are our support in life.
—MARIE VON EBNER-ESCHENBACH

Do you know how to accept support? Or are you so caught up in taking care of everybody else that no one has a chance to take care of you? You tell yourself that you don't want to bother anyone else. Maybe you're really afraid of being dependent or vulnerable, or too proud to accept help from others. Perhaps you don't feel you deserve it. So you turn to food instead.

Chances are the people to whom you've been so much help would love the opportunity to help you, too. They would benefit from the satisfaction of knowing they can be a support. The next time you're feeling down and about to turn to food for comfort, look to a friend, instead, and share your feelings. Practice accepting love as well as giving it.

Support is all around me, but I need to learn to receive it.

I used to think that man must suffer to become strong. But now I think he must have joy to become good. —WILHELM VON HUMBOLDT

Avoid the temptation of playing the martyr and creating a drama around your pain. Hardships are a part of life that we all must endure. Get through those that befall you as well as you can, but don't seek them out. There is no glory in suffering. The real accomplishment is to find joy in life—in good times and bad. Learn how to laugh and live well. Celebrate life through your everyday actions.

Joy is as much a part of life as pain and suffering.

JUNE 27

Who does not carry heaven within himself will seek heaven in vain in all the universe.
— OTTO LUDWIG

Nothing can take the place of self-love and self-acceptance. Sometimes we turn to food to try to fill these needs, but in doing so find that real happiness slips further and further from our reach. Anyone who has ever gorged himself, and then felt awful afterward, knows this.

One way to begin shifting your focus inside, where it belongs, is to start a daily meditation program. Meditate for a few minutes when you awaken in the morning, or at a quiet time during the day. Sit quietly and clear your mind. When thoughts come up let them drift away. Use a mantra such as "om," which you repeat over and over, as a helpful aid.

True happiness and contentment are generated by my own internal spring.

JUNE 28

Good health is probably one of the most important foils. Nothing seems particularly grim if your head is clear and your teeth are clean and your bowels function properly.
— M. F. K. FISHER

Do you know what you need to eat to maintain good health? The USDA food pyramid offers a general daily guideline: several servings each of fruit, vegetables, and whole grains; as well as moderate amounts of dairy, meat, or fish; and minimal fats. Some people feel better when they skip the meat or dairy products. Others have allergies they need to take into account. Teenagers have special needs, as do women of a certain age who need more calcium and iron. What keeps your body in optimum health?

Above all, remember what food is for: It's fuel to keep our bodies in working order. Eat for health, and the rest will follow.

I will contribute to my own good health by eating properly.

Rest has cured more people than all the medicine in the world. —HAROLD J. REILLY

Next time you head for the snack machine or the cupboard for something to boost your energy, ask yourself if what you really need is some extra sleep instead. It's easy to get caught up in taking care of your responsibilities and other people's needs and forget to get the rest your body needs. So you fall into the trap of turning to coffee and other stimulants to keep going.

It's natural for our energy level to ebb and flow during the day. Other cultures recognize this with the mid-afternoon siesta. It may not be possible for you to lie down during the afternoon or at other times when you feel you need rest, but you can do the next best thing. Walk outside if you are in a highrise and take a few minutes to sit quietly next to a fountain or garden. Close your eyes for a minute or two at your desk. If you're at home, take a twenty-minute nap. A short rest can help you resist the temptation to consume food you don't need.

Getting enough rest is part of honoring my body and taking care of my needs.

Self-restraint is feeling your oats without sowing them. —SHANNON FIFE

Temptation strikes—and what do you do about it? You have a choice. You can be overwhelmed by your cravings and give in to them. Or you can acknowledge them, feel them wash over you—and let them pass you by. Try the latter once and see what happens. Be aware of how it feels. Then enjoy the satisfaction of knowing that you resisted the urge to cave in. Try it again. And again. Soon it will be as much a habit as binge eating once was.

I won't deny my cravings, but I won't give in to them, either.

JULY 1

Man lives by habit indeed, but what he lives for is thrills and excitements.

—WILLIAM JAMES

You've changed your eating and exercise habits and now you have a new routine. Congratulations! Keep going, and it will only get easier. You'll eventually get to the point where eating is no longer your major preoccupation.

As you get comfortable following your program, remember to allow yourself some time for spontaneity and unplanned fun. Get away for the weekend with your partner to a place you've never been before. Take up a hobby that stretches you in a new way. Throw a costume party. Now that you're not seeking excitement in unhealthy habits, learn how to find it in other places.

I accept the part of me that needs excitement as well as security.

A simple enough pleasure, surely, to have breakfast alone with one's husband, but how seldom married people in the midst of life achieve it.
—ANNE MORROW LINDBERGH

A quiet meal with your spouse or partner can seem like a luxury in a busy life. Kids, jobs, and gym schedules all compete for our time. We're always running in different directions, it seems. But now and then, we just need to insist on it. Meet at a restaurant if it's too hectic at home.

Time shared together over a meal is invaluable. You're both sitting down and can engage in real conversation. It's not enough just to pass in the halls, sleep together in the same bed, and zone out in front of the TV.

Meals can be a time to nourish my relationships.

We act as though comfort and luxury were the chief requirements of life, when all that we need to make us really happy is something to be enthusiastic about. —CHARLES KINGSLEY

If luxury and comfort were what made us happy, the rich would be the most contented people in the world—and we know this isn't true. What we need instead is something to care about, a passion that gets us up out of bed in the morning with excitement about the day ahead.

What do you really care about? Look to the things you've always been interested in. Is there something you can pursue? What makes you happy today? Can you improve your skills and learn more about it?

It doesn't matter what I care about. It matters that I care about something.

JULY 4

Beyond a wholesome discipline, be gentle with yourself. You are a child of the universe no less than the trees and the stars; you have a right to be here. —MAX EHRMANN

There are so many ways we can be hard on ourselves, and just as many ways to be kind. Why not take the easy path and avoid throwing unnecessary temptations in our way?

We are being good to ourselves when we keep the house stocked with delicious, low-fat foods and leave the junk at the store for someone else. We can be gentle with ourselves by giving ourselves the same understanding and compassion we give to other people.

Like every other living thing on the planet, I deserve to be treated with kindness.

JULY 5

We're all of us sentenced to solitary confinement inside our own skins, for life. —TENNESSEE WILLIAMS

Sometimes we have things on our minds that we can't discuss with anyone else. Perhaps there's no one to talk to confidentially, or we'd rather work it out ourselves. At these times it's often helpful to write our thoughts and feelings down on paper. This allows us to explore our often chaotic emotions in a linear way. Sometimes we find the answer this way, other times it just feels good to express what's in our hearts. A journal can be like a friend that's there for us whenever we feel the burden of our solitude.

Keeping a journal can be inexpensive therapy that teaches me about myself.

One's eyes are what one is, one's mouth what one becomes. —JOHN GALSWORTHY

Be careful of what you take in. If you expose yourself to large doses of violence and junk culture, they're going to become a part of you. Surround yourself with gossip, and it can't help but rub off.

Equally important, watch what comes out when you open your mouth. Are you always putting yourself down or apologizing for yourself? Or do you seize every opportunity to flaunt your successes? Try to find a middle ground.

Character is formed by my everyday actions.

To try to create something worth creating, as our life's work, is the way to understand what joy is in this life. —W. R. INGE

It's time to get your mind off food and onto something else of real importance. Look at all areas of your life: marriage, job, family life, creative endeavors, community involvement. Reevaluate your goals. What do you want to do before you die? Your goals probably won't involve food, but may instead center on learning a new skill, developing a better relationship with your children or spouse, helping someone less fortunate, or reaching a new level in your career.

I will seek out a worthwhile purpose for my life.

The road to wisdom? Well it's plain / And simple to express: / Err / And err / And err again / But less / And less / And less. —PIET HEIN

Everyone slips up. You will too. It's guaranteed. You'll eat the food you told yourself you would avoid. You'll skip an exercise session because you just didn't feel like going.

Instead of beating yourself up (and consoling yourself with a box of chocolates afterward), it's helpful to look at the situation unemotionally: What was the trigger that led to your downfall? Was it lack of sleep? Emotional stress? Boredom at work? Is there something you can do to avoid falling into the same trap next time?

After you've seen what you can learn from the situation, put the mistake behind you and start over again. Sure, you'll trip up again (it's the price of being human) but eventually, if you look at your mistakes as lessons, they'll become less of a problem.

What can I learn from the mistakes I make today?

The best breakfast is a breath of morning air and a long walk. —HENRY DAVID THOREAU

Daily exercise and deep breathing are important habits for all of us to cultivate. Not too long ago exercise was not something you had to seek out—it was a part of your everyday life. You worked hard at a job, at home or on the farm, and you walked most places you went. Today most of us sit for eight hours a day at our jobs and drive rather than walk to reach our destinations.

Today, start the day with a walk in the fresh morning air. You'll get your metabolism going and feel like you've had a moment of peace before the insanity begins. Make this a habit—a half hour of walking each day, more when you have the time and energy. Feel your mood improve, your muscles tone up, and the excess pounds melt away.

Today I will start the day with fresh air and a walk before breakfast.

The porcupine, whom one must handle gloved, may be respected, but is never loved.
—ARTHUR GUITERMAN

Do you take constructive criticism well, or do you respond as though you are being attacked? Do you often feel people are insulting you or talking behind your back? Do you wear your insecurity on your sleeve? Do you try to hold onto the upper hand at all costs?

If you answered yes to these questions, you may be a little difficult to be around at times. Learn to let down the defenses now and then. Fighting every battle to the finish only serves to alienate you from the very people you seek to impress. When you allow your humanity to show through, warts and all, other people feel more comfortable to be themselves, too.

I don't always have to be right.

In extreme youth, in our most humiliating sorrow, we think we are alone. When we are older we find that others have suffered too.
—SUSANNE MOARNY

There's something so humbling and yet so liberating about confessing our darkest secrets to another. We discover in our sharing that, much to our surprise, we are not alone in our experiences. Beneath the placid surface of the ordinary lives around us we find bubbling caldrons of pain and joy in every person. We realize that although we may be completely unique, we are also in many ways the same. We do not struggle under the weight of our burdens alone.

Confessing my secrets can be good for my soul.

Where ambition ends, happiness begins.
—HUNGARIAN PROVERB

Setting goals is an important step toward achievement, but when they become our sole preoccupation, we are in trouble. Always focused on an uncertain future, we fail to enjoy the only thing that is truly ours—the moment that exists right now.

We are not perfect; we may even be highly flawed. But we can't let that stop us from appreciating the one fine quality we have or the one bright spot that exists in an otherwise unremarkable existence. Even as we strive to improve, we can appreciate the goodness that exists today. Otherwise, happiness will continue to elude us, even after we reach our goals.

This moment is priceless, for it is what I have right now.

There is no failure except in no longer trying.
—ELBERT HUBBARD

It ain't over till you stop trying. You can slip up every day, three times a day, but as long as you keep trying you're on the right track. It's when you give up entirely that you're in trouble.

Weight loss is something you know you want badly; in giving up the effort you've given up on yourself. But when you try and fail and try again, you demonstrate your commitment to a better life. So don't get discouraged when you don't meet your goals. Just having a goal is a step in the right direction.

I will keep going, even when I'm tempted to give it all up.

I have never seen a bad television program, because I refuse to. God gave me a mind, and a wrist that turns things off. —JACK PAAR

If you're wasting your time in mindless activities that you don't really enjoy, take action! Turn off the television, take a walk, get involved. We allow a "safe" activity such as watching TV to eat up our hours, and before we know it our lives are passing us by. Time is our most precious gift. Don't let it slip away.

My time is valuable, and I will make the most of it.

If you would cure anger, do not feed it. Say to yourself: "I used to be angry every day; then every other day; now only every third or fourth day." When you reach thirty days offer a sacrifice of thanksgiving to the gods. —EPICTETUS

Anger is one of the appetites that, if we are to be happy and healthy, must be kept in check. Perhaps you never "lose" your temper, or even openly express anger. But does it simmer below the surface when you're caught in traffic, or stuck with a rude salesperson at the department store? Do your friends and family feel it as silent hostility directed at them when they don't meet your expectations?

The answer is not to suppress your anger, but to become aware of it. You always have a choice whether to be angry or not. When someone cuts you off in traffic, you can just as easily forget about it as get mad. People disappoint you when you've set up expectations they never agreed to meet in the first place.

Excessive anger is bad for my health and happiness. I will look at the role it is playing in my life.

Every day one should at least hear one little song, read one good poem, see one fine painting, and—if at all possible—speak a few sensible words. —GOETHE

Spiritual emptiness is an epidemic taking over our society. It's apparent in the problems we see in our youth, the increasing crime rates in our cities and towns, the way we treat each other, and the isolation we feel inside. Finding a cure for this disease sometimes seems futile: How can you battle something so vast and ephemeral, especially in a world that's constantly changing?

The only place to begin is with ourselves, starting with the little things we do each day. We can bring beauty and truth into our world by exposing ourselves to just one work of fine art, an inspired poem, a beautiful song, a thoughtful conversation each day. Taking time for this will enrich our lives and give us more to offer those around us.

I will renew my spirit by taking the time each day to experience art and beauty.

No one with a good hobby is ever lonely for a long time. —BERAN WOLFE, M.D.

There's something invigorating about being around people who have a passion for what they do in their spare time. It doesn't really matter what their hobby is —buying and renovating old houses or collecting rare stamps. They meet other people with the same interest or they share their excitement with observers, and suddenly the energy is multiplied. The enthusiasm they invest is contagious because they care so deeply themselves.

What outside interest am I passionate about in my own life? Is there a hobby I want to pursue?

Few men during their lifetime come anywhere close to exhausting the resources dwelling within them. There are deep wells of strength that are never used. —ADMIRAL RICHARD BYRD

At the point when all seems lost, and you just don't think you can go on, hold on a minute longer. Resist the urge to run to the store for that half gallon of chocolate fudge ice cream.

Each time you reach a difficult point and dig in your heels rather than give in, you draw deeper from the renewable well of strength you carry inside. If you've never drawn on it before, you may not know it's there. But if you let this craving pass you by, you will discover a new reservoir of strength available to you now and in the future. Temptations will become easier and easier to resist.

Food cravings are no match for my inner strength.

JULY 19

All the things I really like to do are either immoral, illegal or fattening.

—ALEXANDER WOOLLCOTT

For the food-obsessed, eating may be the only pleasurable event of the day. If this is true for you, you need to seek out activities that nurture your body in other ways. Spend some time in your garden working with plants and soil. Buy some mineral salts or fragrant oils for your bath and take a long soak once a week. Splurge on a massage once a month, or a regular manicure and pedicure. Join a hiking club with a friend. Expand your horizon of pleasurable activities.

I will open myself up to receive pleasure in activities other than eating.

JULY 20

Life is like playing a violin solo in public and learning the instrument as one goes on.

—SAMUEL BUTLER

Unfortunately, for those of us who seek perfection, there is no dress rehearsal for life. We arrive on stage, the curtain goes up, and the show begins. No time to practice, no time to study the script.

Be gentle with yourself when you stumble or miss a cue. You're doing the best you can do with the information you have. Ask yourself what you can learn to improve your performance next time. It might even turn out that what seems like a mistake now was exactly the right thing to do.

I will let go of my expectations of perfection and be content with doing the best I can.

The riders in a race do not stop short when they reach the goal. There is a little finishing canter before coming to a standstill. There is time to hear the kind voices of friends and to say to one's self, "the work is done."

—OLIVER WENDELL HOLMES, JR.

When friends ask, "Have you lost weight?" and then compliment you on how you look, don't put them off modestly. Look them in the eye and say, "Thank you. Yes, I have."

You've worked hard to reach this point and you've earned your rewards. For so long you've felt bad about how you looked. Part of adapting to the "new you" is to learn how to be comfortable accepting praise and feeling good about yourself.

I will allow myself to enjoy the fruits of my labor.

The toughest thing about success is that you've got to keep on being a success.

—IRVING BERLIN

This is the point that distinguishes the commercial diets, the fad diets, the lose-twenty-five-pounds-before-my-high-school-reunion diets from the real thing.

Because while it's certainly not easy to lose weight, it's an even greater challenge to keep it off. But you're already ahead of the game. You've slowly increased your physical activity, and now daily exercise is part of your life. Your eating habits have changed for the better. You're not on a grapefruit-and-celery or a liquid diet; you've got a balanced diet that you can live with for the rest of your life. You've weaned yourself from the high-sugar, high-fat habit.

Is there anything else I can do to help make my healthy choices a lifetime habit?

Latent in every man is a venom of amazing bitterness, a black resentment; something that curses and loathes life, a feeling of being trapped, of having trusted and been fooled.
— PAUL VALÉRY

Somehow we have interpreted the fairy tales of our youth to mean that life should always treat us fairly. Happy endings are our birthright. Our prince or princess will arrive to sweep us off our feet.

But take a closer reading of those fairy tales and you find them filled with extreme emotions and awful events. The happy endings to these stories are the hopes we all share, but the stories themselves—like life—contain both good and evil. Cinderella is abused by her sisters. Hansel and Gretel are trapped by an old woman who wants to see them dead. As in the fairy tales, life can be anything but fair.

Negativity is a part of our emotional makeup. I don't have to dwell in it, but I will accept its presence.

You can't put the facts of experience in order while you are getting them, especially if you are getting them in the neck. —LINCOLN STEFFENS

Truths about ourselves seem so obvious after we've discovered them. We know that big family events make us nervous and that when we're nervous we overeat. So why did we attend so many family gatherings and eat and eat and eat? Perhaps we stayed in a marriage too long. With each unhappy year came more unwanted pounds. Wasn't it so obvious? Why did we let it go on?

When the room is spinning, we often can't see the door. Turmoil disguises our real feelings. Self-deception can seem like self-preservation in this state.

When the time is right, when we are ready, we sort out the truth. Don't blame yourself for not realizing it earlier. You may not have been able to. Be thankful you've come to it now.

I won't waste time beating myself up for things I wish I had known earlier. There's time to make use of the lessons now.

Every act of creation is first an act of destruction. —PABLO PICASSO

As you slim down and metamorphose into your new self, be prepared to say goodbye to parts of your former life that no longer serve you well: the "fat" clothes you got used to wearing, which kept you hidden from view; the defenses you put up to keep others from getting too close; the bad habits (flawed though they may have been) that have given you some comfort through the years.

You must let go of the things that no longer serve you well to make room for those that will.

Life is a continual dying and rebirth. I am willing to let go.

Every gain made by individuals or society is almost instantly taken for granted.
—ALDOUS HUXLEY

How much have you lost so far? One pound? Ten? Fifty? What improvements have you made in your routines? Have you taken the time to pat yourself on the back for these successes?

We who are always striving for improvement often forget to give ourselves credit when we accomplish our goals. We reach the peak we were seeking, and right away it's on to the next one. This keeps us in a constant state of dissatisfaction, which motivates us for the next goal. Yet it also keeps our opinion of ourselves unnaturally low because we always see ourselves as striving, as opposed to getting there. This can work against us. Don't forget to give yourself credit when it's due.

I will take a moment today to appreciate the good things I have accomplished.

Gratitude is not only the greatest of all the virtues, but the parent of all the others. —CICERO

True wealth is not measured in what we own, but in what we are grateful for. We can have all the possessions in the world, but without gratitude we have nothing—because they mean nothing to us. Conversely, we can be relatively poor on paper, yet be rich with true friends, a comfortable bed, good health, and an optimistic outlook.

When we know how to appreciate what we are given—whether it be a sunny afternoon in winter or a new sapphire ring—we are truly rich. We have learned the value of life.

How much I have to be grateful for when I really examine my life.

Everything tastes better outdoors.
—CLAUDIA RODEN

What is it about eating outside that makes food taste so much better? If you've got the summer doldrums, or even if you don't, take one of your next meals outdoors. The pleasure you get from eating outdoors will add an unexpected spice to your food.

Set up a picnic on the back lawn or at the beach or in a local park. Grill vegetables or fish with just a little bit of oil. Bring a big fruit salad seasoned with mint, a wild rice casserole, or a no-fat black bean chili. Even simple finger foods taste good with blue skies, a light breeze, and warm sun.

I can create a special-occasion meal just by bringing it outdoors.

Life, we learn too late, is in the living, in the tissue of every day and hour.
—STEPHEN LEACOCK

Each trivial decision we make today helps create our future: Shall I have fruit or chocolate cake for dessert tonight? Will I eat my bread plain or with butter? Do I want my salad dressing mixed in or on the side? A successful diet is built on making more right than wrong choices in every hour of every day. Tomorrow has nothing to do with it. Today is where the future is made.

All that I have, all that I am, resides in this moment.

If one begins eating peanuts one cannot stop.
—H. L. MENCKEN

We can train ourselves to eat many high-fat foods in moderation, but some foods it's just easier to avoid. Peanuts, for example.

Consider that each peanut contains nearly half a gram of fat. And how many peanuts in a handful? If you tossed down just twenty, you'd have consumed ten grams of fat. Add to that the temptation most of us have to keep going until we suddenly notice we've finished off a quarter of the can. Is this how you want to spend your fat allowance? Sometimes it's better to keep foods like this out of the house altogether.

There are some foods that spell trouble for a weight-loss program. I will do myself a favor and avoid them.

Every dawn signs a new contract with existence.
—HENRI FREDERIC AMIEL

No matter how many times we trip and falter, we must be prepared to put the past behind us and try again. Over the course of our lives we will make mistakes over and over. Our confidence will flag, our energy will be depleted. But we must go on. What is there to gain by giving up? Certainly we will not reach our goal by stopping, nor will we find peace of mind.

No, the only way to be true to ourselves—good to ourselves—is to take our mark and begin again.

Today I get a fresh start.

AUGUST 1

The experience of strolling by one's self through the vast multitudes of a strange city is one of the most wonderful in life.
—GAMALIEL BRADFORD

Vacations away from home are commonly regarded as the scourge of the dieter. You're eating out a lot, making it harder to control portion size and fat intake. Your routine is disrupted, making it easier to give up all your good habits. Without access to your regular gym or workout classes, exercise often becomes a catch-as-catch-can proposition.

What you can do in self-defense is make exercise a pleasurable part of your travel experience. Skip the tour buses and rental cars and do your sightseeing on foot. There's no better way to get to know a city. Walk to historic sites. Do a tour of museums and churches. Take a stroll through a beautiful neighborhood. Follow your interests. At the end of the day, you can enjoy that special meal without guilt.

I can incorporate exercise into my vacation itinerary.

AUGUST 2

One thing I know: the only ones among you who will be really happy are those who will have sought and found how to serve.
—ALBERT SCHWEITZER

Not all of us are lucky enough to have jobs that allow us to feel as though we're doing some good in the world. And even those of us who enjoy meaningful careers may feel we have talents that cannot be used in our work.

Volunteer work can satisfy that need to serve others that doesn't get met elsewhere. Find an outlet that suits you, one in which you have something special to contribute.

You don't have to feel anonymous and isolated in your community; reach out and make a connection.

Helping other people will improve the quality of my life.

AUGUST 3

For purposes of action nothing is more useful than narrowness of thought combined with energy of will. —HENRI FREDERIC AMIEL

When you keep your eyes focused on your dreams and put solid effort into making them happen, there is almost nothing that can stand in your way.

If you are serious about change, you are definitely going to see success. Congratulate yourself on your concerted efforts. All it takes now is time.

Goal-setting and belief in my abilities combine for success.

AUGUST 4

Things could be worse. Suppose your errors were counted and published every day, like those of a baseball player. —ANONYMOUS

Our diet errors are not necessarily published, but they do register on our hips and thighs everyday. And, of course, there are occasions such as trips to the doctor and the DMV when our weight becomes a matter of public record. Ugh!

Use your own judgment about how often you want to step on the scales. Some people go nuts and weigh themselves half a dozen times a day. This is just part of the obsessive-compulsive behavior you are trying to halt. Still, a scale can function as a legitimate feedback tool reflecting your progress.

I can keep track of my weight loss without getting carried away.

AUGUST 5

It is a mistake to look too far ahead. Only one link in the chain of destiny can be handled at a time. —WINSTON CHURCHILL

If your goal is to eliminate refined sugar and flour, caffeine, and added fat from your diet, you don't necessarily have to take it cold turkey. It may be easier, and more productive, to phase each element out bit by bit. That way your system is not going to go bonkers while it tries to adjust to a whole new set of circumstances. Say you start with the caffeine products, then move on to the refined sugar. All along the way you are trimming fat whenever you can. Eventually you'll get the job done, and it won't have disrupted your life in the process. Not as dramatic, perhaps, but a lot more pleasant.

It may be best for me to take changes one step at a time.

You can put everything, and the more things the better, into salad, as into a conversation; but everything depends upon the skill of mixing.
—CHARLES DUDLEY WARNER

You don't have to limit your salads to the same old standards—iceberg or even romaine. Try some arugula, raddicchio, or radish sprouts for a change. Pick up a good vegetarian cookbook and see what kinds of combinations they recommend. The same with vegetable side dishes and casseroles: Everybody gets bored with carrots and corn after awhile. Expand into cooking with fennel, eggplant and escarole. Try everything in your produce section or farmer's market at least once. Make it a point to experiment and see what else you like.

Whenever I have a little extra time, I will try a new salad or vegetable dish.

Once you say you're going to settle for second, that's what happens to you in life, I find.
—JOHN F. KENNEDY

If you want to lose twenty pounds, don't tell yourself you'll probably only be able to get rid of ten. Go the distance. You can break up your weight-loss program into smaller increments—focusing on five-pound hurdles—to make it more manageable as you are going along. But aim high when you're thinking of your ultimate goal. You're working hard at this anyway, so you might as well be happy with where you end up.

I will aim high and believe in myself. It can be done.

To dare to live alone is the rarest courage; since there are many who had rather meet their bitterest enemy in the field, than their own hearts in the closet. —CHARLES CALEB COLTON

What is it that we are afraid of finding when we keep our own hearts in the closet rather than looking at them in the light? Is it that we believe we are monsters or failures or, perhaps, just empty inside? Or is it that fear has paralyzed us, and we've just become used to keeping that door shut?

What does it mean to you to look into your own heart? Imagine what you will find there and how you will feel. Is there a way you can explore this territory a little at a time so it is less frightening? Is there a wise guide, such as a therapist or religious professional, who can accompany you on the journey?

I may find that the closet is not so scary once I open the door.

We can destroy ourselves by cynicism and disillusion just as effectively as by bombs.
—KENNETH CLARK

Don't let your inner critic destroy your dreams. When you reach a tough challenge in your diet process and those old negative tapes start to kick in, refuse to let them get you down. Those voices that mock you with "you can't" and "you won't" don't have to set you back. Instead, let your newfound confident self stand up to the cynic and disarm her.

Find out where those ugly voices originated in your life and expose them to the light. You may be able to detach yourself from them once and for all. Perhaps they came from bad experiences that you had as a child at school or from an adult who repeated them to you. You can define those voices as relics of a time that is no longer significant to your life.

I don't have to give the critic power over my life.

The more wild and incredible your desire, the more willing and prompt God is in fulfilling it, if you will have it so. —COVENTRY PATMORE

Keep fanning the flames of your desire to improve your life through weight loss. Give yourself pep talks all the time. Repeat positive affirmations throughout the day, particularly when you face temptation. Record your progress—pounds and inches dropped—on a chart that you look at from time to time. Keep your eyes focused on your goal.

The greater my enthusiasm, the easier it will be to keep going.

Give an hour a day to your brain; think—and think regularly every day. An open mind is the best beauty parlor. —FAY WRAY

Cultivate interests outside of dieting. Don't let yourself become dull—a one-note songbird. Just as you've opened your mind to see yourself in a new light, expand your thinking to encompass worlds other than the ones you usually visit. Read up on astronomy, take a language course, join a discussion group, or just sit and ponder awhile.

No matter how attractive a person is, they lose points with most people if they've got nothing going on upstairs.

I can expand my mind as I shrink my waistline.

AUGUST 12

Sweet are the uses of adversity, which, like the toad, ugly and venomous, wears yet a precious jewel in his head. —WILLIAM SHAKESPEARE

"Why me?" we ask ourselves when adversity is thrown our way. We are presuming that trials are regrettable, but we are wrong. Every troubled situation offers us a gift that can be obtained in no other way. There's no more effective teacher than misfortune. With it we learn, we grow, we find a new jewel.

Lord, what I can learn from this trouble?

AUGUST 13

Experience enables you to recognize a mistake when you do it again. —FRANKLIN P. JONES

Have you begun to recognize the common pitfalls that lead you to overeating? Maybe soon you'll even learn to avoid them. Sometimes we get a lesson right away on the first shot. Other times our brains are so obtuse or the habit is so bred into us that it takes repeated occasions—and sometimes years—of stepping into the same trap before we learn how to sidestep it.

But with your motivation so high, all of your learning experiences are accelerated now. You're "getting" things so much faster.

Life is a workshop, and I'm bound to get dirty.

To lengthen thy life, lessen thy meals.
— BENJAMIN FRANKLIN

Medical research indicates that those who eat less tend to live longer. Not only do they have reduced risks of the common life-shortening diseases, it seems that they put less wear and tear on their bodies overall, by not working them so hard with difficult digestion tasks.

But this is no call to starvation; it's still important to eat enough to get the proper nutrition. Find a happy medium. When you cut back, trim out the garbage and sugar and fat. Load up on the foods that are easy on your digestive system.

I will continue to be good to my body by eating lots of fruits, vegetables, and grains.

There is nothing noble about being superior to some other man. The true nobility lies in being superior to your previous self.
— HINDU PROVERB

Comparing yourself to others is like judging the virtues of apples and oranges. Both are fruits, but the resemblance stops there. You're comparing two completely different things. The same is true of us. Though we are human, and may have similarities, we all have our own individual characters. Judging our relative superiority is like asking which is the superior fruit. It depends on the taste of the observer.

My own progress is the only reliable yardstick.

You never find yourself until you face the truth.
— PEARL BAILEY

The longer we delude ourselves about the truth of ourselves, the longer it takes to heal. Do yourself a favor and open your heart to the moment. That's all you have to do. You don't have to force anything, or struggle. It's just a matter of being willing to look. And when you do, it will all become clear. Even your next step will reveal itself in time.

Receptivity is a great teacher.

How beautiful it is to do nothing, and then rest afterward. — SPANISH PROVERB

On a hot summer day there's almost nothing better than a tall glass of something cool to drink and a hammock to stretch out in. When the business world slows down and everyone else is operating on vacation time, you can also take the opportunity to catch up on your relaxation, even if you're not going away. Spend a whole weekend just lolling about, getting up only for long, leisurely walks or an invigorating swim. Reschedule errands and do your laundry later. Get your kids involved in a game of Monopoly, an art project, or computer games that will keep them occupied while you relax, or hire a sitter to watch them and prepare their meals. Relaxation is as important to your health as food and air. Make sure you get your share.

If I don't give myself down time, who will?

Do not wish to be anything but what you are, and try to be that perfectly.
—St. Francis de Sales

Losing weight may be a catalyst for all kinds of changes, but then again, it may not. If your idea of a good time is a two-week backpack trip in the northern Rockies, it's unlikely that you'll turn into a Chanel-suited ingenue after your excess weight is gone. But perhaps you will. Whoever you are, however, it's important to stay true to yourself. Try new experiences, but pay attention to how they make you feel.

I just need to be myself and everything will fall into place.

It is more blessed to give than to receive, so give to yourself as much as you can as often as you can. —LaVerne Porter Wheatley Perry

We hesitate to do things for ourselves, thinking it means we are selfish. It sometimes seems a little silly to buy ourselves a special bouquet of flowers or another kind of treat. But why not do it? We know best what makes us happy. And we are just as deserving of our gifts and kindnesses as anybody else in our lives.

When I give to myself I affirm the beauty of giving.

AUGUST 20

Our life is composed greatly from dreams, from the unconscious, and they must be brought into connection with action. They must be woven together. —ANAÏS NIN

We must have dreams; they are necessary for life. But dreams alone do not carry us through life. We have to learn to convert our dreams into action. Action is a commitment we make to ourselves that says we believe in the value of our dreams and are willing to pursue them.

Throughout our lives, dreams and action continue their dance. One does not exist without the other. They both have their vital place.

I will have the courage to dream and the courage to take action.

AUGUST 21

The world is a looking glass and gives back to every man the reflection of his own face.
—WILLIAM MAKEPEACE THACKERAY

When you're going through a lot of big changes, as you do with weight loss, it's helpful to have a buddy to give you some feedback along the way. Enlist the support of someone who is willing to make herself available to be your sounding board and mirror. It could be someone on a weight-loss program of her own, or perhaps just a good friend who can give you honest feedback. Ask your buddy to tell you about the changes she sees; call her to share the temptations you faced during the day and the triumphs of which you are proud.

Do the same thing for her, whatever her own journey may be.

Following a buddy system can give me invaluable feedback and encourage my progress.

AUGUST 22

Any fool can criticize, and many of them do.
—ARCHBISHOP C. GARBETT

As you shed your physical layer of protection you are apt to feel more exposed. Develop a thick skin to criticism, particularly that which is not offered in a constructive way. Prepare yourself for the reactions you will get from people—good and bad—as they notice your weight loss and the change in your life habits. Some people may feel threatened. It's often the ones who have the least to add to the conversation who say the most. Learn to ignore them and focus inside.

I don't have to let criticisms from others take me by surprise. When they appear, I just let them roll off my back.

AUGUST 23

No one knows what he can do till he tries.
—PUBLILIUS SYRUS

You've increased your exercise and now probably depend on it to boost your energy, keep you in shape, and ease the stress in your life. One year ago, would you have thought you could do what you're doing now?

Maybe you can take yourself further still. Could you be working out a little longer, lifting a little more weight, or adding another workout session to your regimen? It's helpful to reevaluate our routines now and then and see where we might have outgrown them.

What seemed impossible yesterday is easily within my grasp today. Who knows what I may be able to do tomorrow?

If you live alone, offset your solitude by seeing as much of your friends as possible.
— GELETT BURGESS

One of the tough things about keeping up with friends when you're on a weight-loss program is that socializing often revolves around food. Typically, if you want to talk, you're meeting them for dinner, drinks, or dessert.

Instead of always catching up with friends over a meal, get together for exercise instead. Go for a hike or a long walk through the neighborhood and talk along the way. Work out together at the gym and chat in the Jacuzzi afterward. Have a standing arrangement to meet for yoga or an aerobics class once a week. A benefit to working out with friends is that it often keeps us exercising on those days when we would be tempted to shrug it off if we were on our own.

What exercise activities can I share with a friend?

Water is the best of all things. — PINDAR

Our bodies are composed primarily of water, so it makes sense that nutritionists advise us to drink plenty of it. Some say to drink six to eight glasses of water a day, but that's just a rule of thumb. Conditions are different for each person and vary according to the amount our bodies are using up. Generally, dieters need to get plenty, and summer is a good time for everyone to drink a little more. Water keeps us healthy and flushes out our systems. Remind yourself to drink more than you think you need, for most of us don't drink enough. Have a glass of water when you're tempted to snack but aren't truly hungry. Choose water over diet sodas whenever you can. It might seem a little boring at times, but there's no better taste when you're really thirsty.

Water keeps my body functioning well. I'll remember to replenish my supply.

When one friend washes another both become clean. —DUTCH PROVERB

Sharing in the little details of another person's life enriches us in so many ways. In the process of getting to know the other person and sharing ourselves with him or her, we learn things we couldn't have discovered any other way. And no matter who is doing the giving or receiving, both benefit from the close bond of intimacy that is created.

But cultivating a good friend takes effort, time, and commitment, just like everything else that's worthwhile. Why not take some of the energy you used to channel into obsessing about food and use it in the service of developing good friendships? You'll get so much more in return.

I can even talk to a friend about my eating disorder. We both may benefit.

Going slowly does not stop one from arriving. —FULFULDE PROVERB

Patience now, patience! Are you still moving in the right direction? Have you lost a few pounds, quelled some unreasonable cravings, and improved your diet and exercise habits overall? Then congratulate yourself on your progress. It doesn't matter that you haven't lost weight as fast as you would have liked. You're still going to get there eventually.

Maybe you want to cut a little more fat out of your diet, or add another exercise session to your week to stimulate a little more weight loss. That's fine. But stay on a steady keel. Keep your spirits up and banish disappointment. You're doing fine.

It is inevitable that I will reach my goals eventually, as long as I stay on the right path.

AUGUST 28

Every thing that is done in the world is done by hope. —MARTIN LUTHER

Hope is a small seed that we must always protect with our lives. Without hope, everything dies. Hope carries the dreams that all of us have. It gives them shelter, nourishes them in harsh environments, and keeps them alive. It carries the memory of the flowers that come up in the spring and the joy that we will someday feel again. It gives us sustenance to keep on going.

If I have hope I have everything I need.

AUGUST 29

So fresh and exciting this walk up the road with haversack on my back. . . . Off all the wife, the mother, the lover, the teacher, and the violent artist takes over. I am alone. I belong to no one but myself. I mate with no one but the spirit. I own no land, have no kind, no friend or enemy. I have no road but this one.
—SYLVIA ASHTON-WARNER

Now and then, we all need to let go of our obligations, say goodbye to our loved ones, and veer off on our own paths.

It can mean taking a day off for a long, meditative walk in the woods or a relaxing visit to a health spa. Or it can be claiming a whole year for ourselves in which to pursue our own interests instead of tending to other people's.

Either way, we take time to focus on our own needs. We see ourselves in our own orbits, instead of just revolving around other people. We invite our hidden selves to appear and teach us what we need to know.

Some days belong just to me.

AUGUST 30

A man's palate can, in time, become accustomed to anything. —NAPOLEON I

Remember how anemic nonfat foods tasted when you first switched over to them? Now you're so used to them that the old fat-loaded products taste too rich. You've become used to a new way of eating.

What else in your diet needs to be changed? Are you still eating too much sugar? Or sucking down diet drinks and artifically sweetened foods? Maybe you could adjust your palate to do without so much sweet flavor. You've already made major changes. Another adjustment is also within your grasp.

With enough motivation, I can adjust to almost anything.

AUGUST 31

Giving is storing up for oneself.
—NDEBELE PROVERB

Many of us are tempted to overeat when we are feeling physically vulnerable and stressed—when our finances are strained, our jobs are insecure, or our environments seem unstable.

One thing you can do to help yourself until you are able to improve the situation is to go to your friends for support. If you've been giving friendship to them, helping them, supporting them all along, you should feel comfortable turning to them when you need help yourself. Giving is a two-way street. Don't be afraid to ask for what you need when it's your turn.

Good friends are an insurance policy for troubled times.

SEPTEMBER 1

Conditions are never just right. People who delay action until all factors are favorable are the kind who do nothing.

—WILLIAM FEATHER

Today you're in too much of a rush to eat right. Tomorrow you have a big business dinner. The day after that you don't feel well when you wake up so you skip your morning workout.

Excuses for not following your weight-loss program can be never ending. Nothing is ever just quite right when you're performing a task you believe to be unpleasant. You must proceed anyway, in the face of obstacles.

Avoid the dramatic action. Just do whatever you can, when you can. You're better off doing something small toward your goal than doing nothing at all.

This moment is as perfect as it is going to get.

SEPTEMBER 2

Only the person who has faith in himself is able to be faithful to others. —ERICH FROMM

What advice would you give to yourself if you were your friend? What words of encouragement would you offer? What faith in your abilities would you profess?

We reserve these acts of kindness for others and neglect to offer them to ourselves. But if we are willing to neglect ourselves, we will eventually let others down too. We must have faith in ourselves before we can be counted on to be faithful to others.

There are so many things I take on faith. Why not this?

SEPTEMBER 3

There is less leisure now than in the Middle Ages, when one-third of the year consisted of holidays and festivals. —RALPH BORSODI

So much of our time is consumed by work, work, work. Even our leisure is filled with work and obligations. We have to rebel now and then, loosen the shackles that bind us, and turn ordinary days into holidays. We can do it informally so that we don't create even more work for ourselves. It can be as simple as turning an ordinary party into a scavenger hunt or an everybody-cooks event (hire an industrious teenager to help you clean up afterward.) You can organize your children and their friends into producing a play for the neighborhood on their vacation, or putting on a makeshift circus in somebody's backyard. There are a million ways to bring a more festive air to our daily routines.

As I cultivate my imagination, my daily life grows richer.

Always do one thing less than you can do.
— BERNARD BARUCH

Some people are prone to overextending themselves and subsequently suffer from exhaustion most of the time. The special danger for dieters is that the stress of always doing too much can tip them over into nervous eating as a way to compensate.

You don't owe anybody anything for your existence. Having a cadre of people who "need" you is not much consolation when you're unhappy with the way you look and feel because you're fat. So give yourself room to relax; schedule it in. Just as it's best to allow an extra fifteen minutes for traffic slow-downs when driving to an important appointment, it's a good rule of thumb to figure out how much you can do, and then subtract from there. This should give you the peace of mind to enjoy everything more.

Quantity does not necessarily mean quality.

One cannot think well, love well, sleep well, if one has not dined well. — VIRGINIA WOOLF

In your enthusiasm for losing weight, try not to get carried away and start to eliminate meals. If you're not feeling very hungry, just eat smaller portions—but eat something. Keep yourself nourished with a balanced diet so you have enough energy to thrive.

You want to avoid going after the diet "high" that you sometimes get when you starve yourself and feel so self-righteous, because the other end of the spectrum is the diet "low" that inevitably follows. Suddenly your empty stomach calls out for all those meals it missed, and an out-of-control eating binge is well on its way.

I will give my body the nourishment it needs every day.

SEPTEMBER 6

The kitchen is a good apothecarie's shop.
—WILLIAM BULLEIN

After spending a couple of decades eating cardboard convenience foods and cooking all the value out of vegetables, we're finally rediscovering the medicinal properties of a well-prepared meal. No amount of nutritional supplements, we're finding, can equal the benefit of getting our vitamins and minerals from natural foods. Ideas we once dismissed as old wives' tales—garlic keeping away a cold, chicken soup aiding in recovery—are now being backed up by scientific findings.

How much of the food you eat today will offer you nutrition beyond mere calories?

My kitchen is also my medicine cabinet if I eat properly.

SEPTEMBER 7

The only people who never fail are those who never try. —ILKA CHASE

Our society holds powerful prejudices about people who are overweight or out of shape. Excess weight is typically viewed as the result of sloth, laziness, and a lack of pride.

But in reality, the obese person may instead have impossibly high standards that no one could possibly attain. Rather than face failure, the perfectionist gives up before she begins.

To escape this trap, we can view a weight-loss program not as a test of our character or will, but as an experiment. We will keep trying, experimenting, until we find an approach that works.

I am not afraid of failing because I know I will continue trying until I reach my goal.

In general, mankind, since the improvement of cookery, eats twice as much as nature requires.
— BENJAMIN FRANKLIN

If you've been overeating for years, it may take a little experimentation to find out how much or how little food you need to maintain your ideal weight.

Don't let someone else dictate the terms of your diet; you need to find out how much is right for you. Get into the habit of leaving something on your plate at the end of each meal, particularly if you did not choose the portion size yourself. If you're served more than you know you can or should eat, ask for a doggie bag and put the extra aside right away to eat at a later meal.

The goal is that you eat to satisfy your hunger, no more and no less.

I may find I can eat a lot less food than I'm used to and still leave the table feeling comfortably full.

Do not be anxious about tomorrow; tomorrow will look after itself. — MATTHEW 6:34

As much as we know intellectually that worry does not do us any good, we need to remind ourselves of this from time to time. Worry appears unexpectedly. It registers at such an unconscious level that sometimes we can fret an hour or a day away without realizing it.

So how can you stop worry? Simply by sending it away when you notice it has visited itself in your mind. Refuse to negotiate with it; do not allow it to stay. Worry only wastes our time, and we've wasted enough time already.

I will pay attention to my thoughts today to see if worry is slipping in unnoticed.

The future is not in the past; it is in the future.
—JEAN GUITTON

It is so easy to get locked into believing that the past determines our future. Instead of *having* a history, we think we *are* our histories: "I have been overweight. I will always be overweight."

But just because you have been overweight does not mean you are sentenced to a lifetime of the same. The future does not have to follow the past. One sharp turn of the wheel today, and tomorrow you can be traveling in a completely new direction.

Every day I have an opportunity to rewrite my destiny.

Don't be afraid of opposition. Remember, a kite rises against, not with, the wind.
—HAMILTON MABIE

Many dieters tell stories of friends and family who tried to sabotage their weight-loss efforts. The friends complained that they were getting too thin; spouses worried aloud that they were going to stray. You must learn to let other people's fears bounce off you and not deter you from reaching your goal. Have a talk with them if you want, or just ignore the comments.

Everyone fears change. When your intimates get some experience dealing with the "new" you, their worries will probably become less pronounced.

I will stay true to my own vision and goals.

SEPTEMBER 12

Americans can eat garbage, provided you sprinkle it liberally with ketchup, mustard, chili sauce, tabasco sauce, cayenne pepper, or any other condiment which destroys the original flavor of the dish. —HENRY MILLER

The right condiments can enhance a dish, but there are two requirements. First, the dish itself must be fresh and of the highest quality. Second, the sauce must be the same. A sauce or a seasoning should not serve to drown out bad flavors, rather it should work to enhance those that are already pleasing. Slopping on the goop so that you can stomach a meal constitutes a lack of self-respect.

Garbage goes in cans, not in my stomach.

SEPTEMBER 13

The unendurable thing, to be sure, the really terrible thing, would be a life without habits, a life which continually required improvisation.
—FRIEDRICH NIETZSCHE

As you're shedding bad habits, replace them with good ones. Don't leave important priorities to chance; build them into your routine. Design the life you want to lead.

For example, how many times a week do you want to exercise, and when? If you decide to work out Monday through Thursday mornings for forty-five minutes each day, schedule those times in on your calendar. Make exercise part of a set routine that you don't have to think about and would have to make a real effort to change.

Routines are good when they keep me doing the right thing.

There is no wealth to compare with health of body. —ECCLESIASTICUS 30:16

Let's imagine you have a closet full of fabulous clothes, an expensive car in the driveway and a financial portfolio brimming with prime investments. And to top it all off, you're at your dream weight. If you can't get out of bed because you are chronically ill, does it really matter?

When you're tempted to jump on the bandwagon of fad dieting, or when you're careless with diet pills or medications, remember what it's like to be sick and unable to function. Protect your health; don't take it for granted. Guard it like the treasure it is.

Good health is the foundation of everything I possess.

To err is human, to forgive divine.
—ALEXANDER POPE

To this quotation you could add, "To ask for forgiveness, better still."

Are there wrongs you have committed against another, or angry words you have spoken and later regretted? Sometimes the best thing you can do for yourself is to confess your errors and ask for forgiveness. You may find the other person wasn't even aware of anything you did wrong—or perhaps it has always bothered him. No matter what his feeling about it, the act of confessing is what's vital.

We can be held back by mistakes that weigh heavily on our hearts. Until these past actions are confessed and cleared away, part of us is unable to move ahead.

Do I need to make amends for anything in my past?

SEPTEMBER 16

The man who covets is always poor.
— CLAUDIAN

No matter how slender you are, there are some things you wish for that can never be. Maybe it's the shape of your hips, or the length of your waist, or the way your upper arms look when you wear sleeveless tops. Whatever it is, you want it to be different; you want to look like so-and-so who has the perfect body part in spades.

If you carry these obsessions along with you on your dieting journey, you will always fall short of success. You will never truly be able to look at yourself and appreciate what you are.

You have many fine points; give up the longing and learn to appreciate them!

I will learn how to highlight my strengths and minimize my weaknesses.

SEPTEMBER 17

If you want to be loved, be lovable. — OVID

When it comes to love and affection, we often maintain an "equal giving" policy. We'll give as much as we get, nothing more.

But to increase the amount of love in our lives, we must invest more, too. The more we give, the more we get, for love begets love.

Love that is not given is wasted.

It is common sense to take a method and try it. If it fails, admit it frankly and try another. But above all, try something.
—FRANKLIN D. ROOSEVELT

To avoid letting our setbacks get the best of us, we have to learn to detach them from emotional judgments about our self-worth. Your goal in experimenting with weight-loss methods is to get the job done, not to proclaim yourself a winner or a loser in the game of life.

I will concentrate on getting the job done and stick with what works.

All happiness depends on courage and work.
—HONORÉ DE BALZAC

It's tempting to look for shortcuts to weight loss, but what we lose depends on one simple condition: that we burn off more fat and calories than we consume. There's just no way around it. That's what it takes.

We can make the process as pleasant as possible, but it's still going to be a lot of work. It takes courage and effort to change our habits, to say no to temptations, and to get ourselves moving again. But the effort will pay off; there are rewards waiting for us along the way.

I will get a great amount of satisfaction from achieving my goal.

Food, one assumes, provides nourishment, but Americans eat it fully aware that small amounts of poison have been added to improve its appearance and delay its putrefaction. —JOHN CAGE

It's crept up on us slowly, this poisoning of our food supply. We've been sweet-talked into allowing our foods to be infused with potentially harmful chemicals by the pesticide producers, food manufacturers, and chemical-additive makers who profit from their use. But the distressing effects on our rivers and fields and wildlife are convincing many of us that their gains are not worth our losses.

We know that if manufacturers can devise harmful chemicals to "improve" their products, they also possess the creativity, expertise, and technology to come up with safer alternatives. We can encourage them in this endeavor by the way we spend our money. We can purchase products that are organic and free of harmful chemicals, even if they cost a little more. It may be worthwhile to spend more for these now (the prices will go down as more people buy them) than to pay less for something that destroys our irreplaceable natural resources.

I will show respect to my body and the world I live in by choosing products that are truly healthful and beneficial.

It is one thing to be tempted, another thing to fall. —WILLIAM SHAKESPEARE

"Danger zone" dishes are different for each person—for one it could be crème brûlée, for another eggplant Parmigiana. The commonality is that they are high in fat or sugar and hard to resist overeating once we begin.

Some people find it easier on a weight-loss program to avoid their "dangerous" foods completely. Rather than risk triggering a binge, they avoid the food until they are in better control of their eating compulsions.

But what if the thing you crave is served to you one night, and you do give in? Is all lost for that week's weight loss? It doesn't have to be. Eat slowly, savor the food, and think about what it is that makes it so psychologically powerful to you. Keep asking yourself, "Have I had enough yet?" Stop when the answer is yes. You can change a pattern anytime you want, and this may be your opportunity.

Enough may be just two bites instead of my usual twenty.

SEPTEMBER 22

It is best in the theatre to act with confidence no matter how little right you have to it.
—LILLIAN HELLMAN

Even if you have to resort to playacting, approach your weight loss with confidence. Be confident with yourself and act self-assured with others. Hold the attitude that you just *know* you're going to lose all that extra weight. It's a given. *Of course* you turn down that piece of pie, because you're committed to your weight-loss program. Act as though you have already been successful, even if you're still in the early stages. Create a positive buzz about the progress of your diet so that you'll be surrounded by people who believe you can do it. Then follow it up with action!

I can help make something happen by believing it is so.

SEPTEMBER 23

I've been overweight since I was four. I don't want to overinflate my role and my job, but isn't there more to me than what I weigh?
—JACK NICHOLSON

Famous actors face more pressure to stay slim than most. Their livelihoods depend on it. But all of us live in a world where people are judged by how closely their appearance conforms to current fashion. And so we turn the magnifying glass on ourselves. We imagine that our fat is all that people see when they look at us. But we are more than the sum of our body parts.

Our physical appearance is just one aspect of who we are and what we have to offer. We are individuals with many aspects—not just physical, but mental, emotional, and spiritual. As we present ourselves that way to other people, eventually they will get the picture too.

I am not my body. My body is only a part of me.

Sour, sweet, bitter, pungent, all must be tasted.
—CHINESE PROVERB

Just because you're cutting back on your fat and calorie intake doesn't mean your diet has to be reduced as well. In the totality of world cuisines there are an enormous variety of foods, recipes, and ingredients available to you. Many feature tastes and flavors you may never have encountered.

Out of convenience and habit you may be restricting your diet to a mere fraction of what's available. Why not go in the other direction and expand the variety of foods you eat? Substitute pungent flavor for the excessive fat you used to consume. Stimulate your taste buds with a food that is pleasantly sour or bitter. If you live in a city with different ethnic groups you can easily sample foods in restaurants that incorporate a wide range of flavors. Just ask the waiter to recommend dishes that are low in fat or could be prepared without it. Expand your eating universe!

Seeking out a healthier diet can open up new worlds to me.

Temptation rarely comes in working hours. It is in their leisure time that men are made or marred. —W. M. TAYLOR

It may be easy to resist the snacking urge at work, where you're usually running around or answering phones or working on deadline projects. But at home, well, that's another story. Even when you're busy, temptation lurks nearby in a kitchen cupboard. Outside the home, leisure activities—dinners, drinks, picnics, parties—can easily revolve around food.

You can minimize the potential dangers of leisure-time noshing with a little planning. Keep your cupboards stocked with nonfat snacks: air-popped popcorn, fat-free crackers and cookies, fresh fruit or canned fruit with minimal added sugar, pretzels, and presliced vegetables. Take a nonfat snack with you to events where you might be tempted to indulge in bad-news foods. Give yourself some heathful options.

I am not perfect, but I can work around my weaknesses.

I can enjoy feeling melancholy, and there is a good deal of satisfaction about being thoroughly miserable; but nobody likes a fit of the blues. Nevertheless, everybody has them; notwithstanding which, nobody can tell why. There is no accounting for them. You are just as likely to have one on the day you have come into a large fortune as on the day after you have left your new silk umbrella on the train.

—JEROME K. JEROME

No matter that blue moods come and go throughout our lives. When we're in the grips of one, it feels as though it will never end. But we know it will; it always does. It may take a few hours or a few days, but eventually the mood lifts and we return to a more hopeful state. So ride it out and be easy on yourself while it lasts. Resist the urge to drown it out with food or drink, which will only make you feel worse. (If a mood lasts much longer than a few days, or if you are tempted to do yourself or someone else harm, by all means seek professional help.)

Blue moods are part of life's landscape. They too will pass.

to be nobody but yourself—in a world which is doing its best, night and day, to make you everybody else—means to fight the hardest battle which any human being can fight, and never stop fighting. —E. E. CUMMINGS

You aren't losing weight for your doctor or your husband or your children or your lover or your mother or your friends or your co-workers or the good-lookers at the bar. You are losing weight for yourself.

Ask yourself what you really want out of this deal. What is your motivation and what will keep you going when things get tough?

You're the person who knows what you really need to lose and the best way to do it. Educate yourself, of course, so that you know your health risks and allergies and the most up-to-date diet information. But once you've got that down, trust your instincts. They'll tell you what you need to do.

I'm doing this for me.

Not to know is bad; not to wish to know is worse.
—NIGERIAN PROVERB

If you're not losing weight as fast as you think you should be, maybe there's something you don't know. Perhaps you're eating more than you realize and exercising less than you think.

Try keeping a diet and exercise diary for several days. Write down everything you eat, including all of the nibbles, snacks, and full meals. Jot down a record of your workouts, noting total exercise time and level of strenuousness.

How does it add up? Are there any surprises you were reluctant to admit to yourself? Is there anything you need to alter to get yourself on the proper course?

Knowing is better than not knowing. It's the only way I will realize my dreams.

It is easier to fill a glutton's belly than his eye.
—THOMAS FULLER

The all-you-can-eat salad-bar restaurant can be a dangerous place for a dieter. The food is laid out before us as at a king's banquet, and one low price buys all. Common sense flees out the door, and, in its place, the glutton's eye takes over. We easily fill our plates. Yards and yards of salads coated in rich dressings stretch before us, and that's just the beginning. Thick breads, creamy soups, puddings, entrées—and yet all of it falls under the rubric of "healthy." We know in our hearts it can't really be a low-fat meal, but we allow ourselves to be deceived. In actuality, we're probably consuming more fat and calories than at a traditional roadside steak house.

Keep your wits about you the next time you visit one of these establishments and think about what you are eating. Remember there's no such thing as a free lunch.

Even though a large salad-bar meal may seem like a bargain, I will pay for it in extra pounds.

Autumn is the bite of a harvest apple.
— CHRISTINA PETROWSKY

One of the pleasures of eating fresh produce is the connection it gives us to the changing seasons. If autumn is the bite of a harvest apple, spring is the sampling of the first strawberries and asparagus. Winter is the rediscovery of root vegetables: carrots and potatoes. Summer is a cornucopia of fresh fruits and vegetables: peaches, plums, cherries, and corn on the cob.

To every thing its season. By following these ancient cycles, we find ourselves in sync with the natural world around us.

Each season bears new fruit. I will appreciate what each has to offer.

OCTOBER 1

Art is a mystery. When I start a picture, I don't know no more what I'm going to do than you do.
—MINNIE JONES EVANS

Before the act of creation, every painter faces an empty canvas. What will she do with it? Often she doesn't know until she gets started and the painting begins to emerge.

If we want something new to develop in our lives, we must have the courage to clear out our cluttered minds and live with the emptiness for awhile. We have to toss out old ideas and preconceptions that are no longer of use to us and are just taking up space. Finally, when we have let go of our expectations, there is room for inspiration to appear.

Plans and goals can take us a long way, but sometimes an open mind is what we need most.

OCTOBER 2

Adversity is the state in which a man most easily becomes acquainted with himself, being especially free from admirers then. —SAMUEL JOHNSON

How have your friends reacted to the changes you are going through? If you're lucky, you've got many friends backing you in this endeavor. But there may be others who are annoyed by your new attitudes or resentful that they never see you anymore. If you find some of these friends dropping out of your life for awhile, it's probably all right. As time passes, both of you will adjust to the changes. In the meantime, use the time you have alone, free from peer pressure, to take a closer look at your life.

I can turn this time into an opportunity for reflection.

OCTOBER 3

Man cannot be uplifted; he must be seduced into virtue. —DON MARQUIS

We can tell ourselves over and over again that losing weight and staying fit is good for our health. Right. That incentive may work for some of us, some of the time, but most of us need something a little more enticing to get us through the hard work of weight loss.

Visualize a reward for yourself that would make all this worthwhile. Maybe it's that teeny, tiny black dress you'll be able to fit into soon or the prospect of finally being able to beat your tennis partner on the court. When you are tempted to overeat or skip exercise, conjure up these images. Seduce yourself into sticking to your program.

Something wonderful awaits me after I meet my weight-loss goal.

Music comes first from my heart, and then goes upstairs to my head where I check it out.
—ROBERTA FLACK

While some people seek out every self-improvement program that comes their way, others struggle even to talk about how they feel with a close friend. If you aren't one to verbalize your feelings, find another way to express them. Do you have an affinity for a particular art form—painting, singing, or dancing? You don't have to be a professional to be able to communicate emotion in a dance or a song. In fact, you don't even have to perform them for anyone else. Letting your feelings rise to the surface for your own awareness and enjoyment is enough.

I can express my emotions in many different ways, even channeling them into art.

Work and love—these are the basics. Without them there is neurosis. —THEODOR REIK

If work and love are the twin towers of mental health, you would do well to cultivate the presence of both in your life. They don't have to fall under the traditional definitions. Work can be many things, from homemaking to a corporate job to volunteer tasks. Love doesn't necessarily mean the romantic variety; it can be the love of a child, of a friend, of God.

Work and love offer balance to my life.

Cheerfulness and contentment are great beautifiers, and are famous preservers of youthful looks.
— CHARLES DICKENS

When you're feeling fully alive and happy inside, your inner beauty shines through and gives your face a special glow. When gloominess drags you down, that light is extinguished and some of the beauty seems to dull and fade.

That's why every beauty routine must involve care of the spirit as well as the skin. Beauty is not just skin deep, it emanates from within us.

The light inside me illuminates my beauty.

We glorify rugged wills; but the greatest things are done by timid people who work with simple trust. — JOHN LA FARGE

It is not necessary to be a superhuman individual to achieve a goal such as weight loss. Dropping pounds is not the impossible task we sometimes make it out to be. It is something we can do no matter how weak our willpower and personal strength.

As we step out of our own way and give in to God, we easily return to a healthy state of being. By trusting in the eternal force that powers all of the universe, we know that we, too, can find our balance. We don't have to work so hard; we just need to hold onto our faith. It is well within our reach.

God gives me everything I need.

OCTOBER 8

All human beings need at times to escape from the serious situation in which they find themselves—often just for the joy ride, at times for sanity. —LEON WHIPPLE

When was the last time you spent the whole day just doing something fun? Has it been too long? Well, then it's time for some play: no errand-running, bill-paying, or picking up around the house allowed.

Take the day off and have some fun. Drive your kids to a water park and join in the fun on the slides. Rent a video camera and shoot a mini-movie about your life. Lure a good friend out for window-shopping at some of the more expensive stores in town. Hijack your husband for a romantic tête-à-tête at a local hotel.

Playtime is just as important as work. There's always enough time to have fun.

OCTOBER 9

It is solved by walking. —LATIN PROVERB

It's amazing how many times solutions come to us while we're taking a walk. Or just after we return from one. You are puzzling over a problem, take a walk to clear your head, and boom, there is the answer.

Maybe the extra blood circulation to the brain accounts for it, or maybe it's the result of relaxing your concentration. Whatever it is, use it to your advantage. The next time you are stuck on a problem, take a short walk. You may gain a new insight along the way or, at the very least, you will get some good exercise.

I will take a walk every time I get the chance.

OCTOBER 10

You grow up the day you have your first real laugh—at yourself. —ETHEL BARRYMORE

Continue to laugh at yourself when the occasion for it arises. Loosen up and let your playful side appear. Other people will be attracted by your newfound good humor. When you find you're starting to get too serious, keep it all in perspective with a good joke on yourself that others can enjoy.

Being able to laugh at myself requires a level of self-confidence that makes other people feel at home.

OCTOBER 11

Silence is the door of consent. —BERBER PROVERB

Finding our voices and defining ourselves as individuals means learning to say no. It might start with saying no to a meal and grow to saying no to being treated poorly. Eventually, it could extend into the larger political world. Once you open a new door, who knows where it will lead?

Saying no means setting boundaries. I must learn to do this to feel comfortable with my slimmer self.

OCTOBER 12

Courage is sustained . . . by calling up anew the vision of the goal. —A. G. SERTILLANGES

It may never be easy to continue on a weight-loss program, but by now it should be easier than it was at the start. For one thing, you are closer to your goal. And you've changed your eating habits.

If your commitment starts to flag, review your goals and progress so far. Pull out those clothes you want to fit back into and imagine the life you will lead at your ideal weight. Remember what it is that has kept you going so far. It can continue to carry you to the end.

The reward awaiting me makes the task worthwhile.

OCTOBER 13

The strong man meets his crisis with the most practical tools at hand. They may not be the best tools but they are available, which is all-important. He would rather use them, such as they are, than do nothing. —RAYMOND CLAPPER

One of the tools that serves you well on a weight-loss program is common sense. With it you can figure out how to take care of yourself and sense when you've gone too far or not far enough. There are other useful tools too: patience, persistence, and a flexible mind. And don't forget self-respect.

Qualities such as rock-solid willpower and an abiding faith are what many dieters dream of, but few possess. Lucky you, if you've got those in your kit.

But to complete your task you can improvise, using whatever tools you have at your disposal. Your effort may not be perfect, but it will be adequate to get the job done.

I possess everything I need to complete my task.

She who conceals her disease cannot expect to be cured. —ETHIOPIAN PROVERB

We're ashamed of the way we handle food and so we hide the fact that we have an eating disorder. Bulimia is our own dirty secret. We won't listen when concerned friends confront us about being anorexic—can't they see we're still too fat? And so we pretend to eat to keep them quiet, while secretly we are still starving and purging ourselves to an early grave.

If you're reading this book, you've probably already admitted to having a problem—but have you turned to others yet for help? A nutritionist or family doctor is a logical first step. Family members may be helpful, but if not, think of a friend who might be. If there is no one else, or even if there is, turn to a trained therapist or a group such as Overeaters Anonymous. The problem is bigger than you are right now. It's time to share your burden and get some help.

In my heart, I know when I am in trouble. I will swallow my pride and admit that I need help.

OCTOBER 15

The human soul needs actual beauty even more than bread. —D. H. LAWRENCE

Don't forget to allow time for nature breaks. We need some contact with plants, animals, birds, water—natural beauty—every day. We can go for a walk in the morning before work, or use a lunch break to sit on a park bench or near a fountain during the day. Promise yourself a day or weekend trip out of the city every month or two. There's nothing like breathing in fresh mountain air or walking barefoot on a beach to renew the spirits. We can get blinded by concrete and crime statistics, but nature is a healing force.

Nature's beauty can nourish my spirit.

OCTOBER 16

No diet will remove all the fat from your body because the brain is entirely fat. Without a brain you might look good, but all you could do is run for public office. —COVERT BAILEY

Don't get so carried away with your weight loss that you lose your head *and* your sense of humor! It is possible to go too far.

With your infatuation with your new trim body, don't forget to shower a little attention on your brain too. Keep up with current affairs and read a substantial book regularly. Don't turn the mind-body split into a feast or famine affair—yesterday the mind, today the body.

Is it time to stop losing weight and start concentrating on maintenance?

OCTOBER 17

Joy is everywhere; it is in the earth's green covering of grass; in the blue serenity of the sky; in the reckless exuberance of spring; in the severe abstinence of grey winter; in the living flesh that animates our bodily frame.
—RABINDRANATH TAGORE

The most mundane details of our lives are sometimes the things that give us the most pleasure. What are the things that give you joy? What are you grateful for today? The bird that sings every morning so beautifully from your backyard tree? The crayon masterpiece your son drew for you yesterday? A tender kiss, unexpected, from your lover today?

Write them down. Give a prayer of thanks. Appreciate the many gifts you receive every day; don't let them slip by unnoticed.

My life is blessed with many sources of joy and beauty.

OCTOBER 18

Anxiety is a thin stream of fear trickling through the mind. If encouraged, it cuts a channel into which all other thoughts are drained.
—ARTHUR SOMERS ROCHE

Anxiety is contagious. When it appears in your mind, it quickly spreads to every thought you have. Though it may start as a simple worry, it soon leapfrogs to bigger issues. Soon you are questioning your very being and existence.

Pay attention to those nagging little doubts or unrealistic fears when they are in the early stages. Call up a good friend and get another view. She may be able to help you put things in perspective and banish the anxiety before it eats away at your core.

I have to take charge of my thoughts and not let them be controlled by anxious fears.

OCTOBER 19

I always believed that if you set out to be success-ful, then you already were.
—KATHERINE DUNHAM

This is the kind statement, the one that gives us the benefit of the doubt. It's saying that just trying is a victory in itself. And isn't it? In that one affirmative action of setting out to be successful, we have successfully stared down fear and cynicism. We have made a positive choice.

Learning to aim for success is an achievement in itself.

OCTOBER 20

It is one of the beautiful compensations of this life that no one can sincerely try to help another without helping himself.
—CHARLES DUDLEY WARNER

Intellectual or emotional myopia is some-times a side effect of obesity. Those who are overweight become so focused on themselves and their flaws that they fail to see the larger world around them.

One of the best ways to look be-yond your own troubles is to help some-one else. Seeing the world through an-other's eyes helps to put things into better perspective. And being able to im-prove someone else's life a little does much toward improving your own.

When I can I will look beyond myself to help other people.

How does one kill fear, I wonder? How do you shoot a spectre through the heart, slash off its spectral head, take it by the spectral throat?
— JOSEPH CONRAD

How do we account for the sudden appearance of fear, when it just as quickly ducks away? It shows up like any other passing emotion, fickle and often untrustworthy.

But sometimes fear is quite useful— it's like a yapping dog that warns us of danger outside. Other times it's the unreal product of paranoia and imagination. Most of the fear you encounter in dieting is this latter type; occasionally it is the former. Do you know how to separate these in your mind?

Fear may serve a purpose, but it can also cripple me.

I felt a continual sensation of craving for something, I didn't know what. It was so continual that it seemed an inherent part of life to be hungry, to feel a perpetual irritation of desire—never to be able to rest in contentment and peace.
— KATHARINE BUTLER HATHAWAY

What is it that keeps us so hungry, so restless inside? Is it a longing for a more intense experience of living? Is it dissatisfaction with ourselves and the choices we have made?

We can try to satisfy this restlessness with food. We can let it make us powerfully unhappy. Or we can allow the internal irritant to be a positive force that keeps us striving for something more than a mediocre life. It can be like the proverbial sand in the oyster that creates a pearl—or a life with more meaning.

My spiritual hunger can serve a positive end.

OCTOBER 23

A little with quiet is the only diet.
—GEORGE HERBERT

Your meals may often be noisy affairs, with kids and crowds and clattering dishes. But when you're on a reducing diet, try to minimize some of the distractions when you eat. The overstimulation of a loud dining area may encourage you to eat more because it's hard to concentrate on the food. The noise may also be a symptom of a larger problem—a life that is completely out of your control.

Give yourself room to focus on your eating. You don't have to eat like a monk forever, but try it for awhile right now.

I can ask my family to help me with this experiment.

OCTOBER 24

It is a good rule to face difficulties at the time they arise and not allow them to increase unacknowledged. —EDWARD W. ZIEGLER

Is there a rough spot that you encounter in your life and never quite seem able to leap over? Perhaps there is a mental roadblock holding you back. Best to explore the situation as soon as possible. If you don't, you'll just return to it again and again. And the problem will possibly grow in size.

Time ticks away while you stall.

I have the courage to face my difficulties straight on.

OCTOBER 25

Ten thousand flowers in spring, the moon in autumn, a cool breeze in summer, snow in winter. If your mind isn't clouded by unnecessary things, this is the best season of your life. —WU-MEN

Even at those times when everything seems to be crashing down on us, we still have the haunting beauty of the autumn moon. Winter can bring a flood of unwanted family obligations, but we can appreciate the perfect quiet of falling snow. We can clear our minds of worry so that we can see the thousands of flowers in bloom in the spring. And we can walk in the summer twilight and savor the sensation of the cool breeze blowing through our hair.

Even if life were to give us nothing else to enjoy, these would be amazing gifts. But we have so much more. We just need to learn to see through the haze of distractions to the beauty that exists in our lives.

Every day brings new miracles if I only can see them.

OCTOBER 26

It is not the horse that draws the cart, but the oats. —RUSSIAN PROVERB

Give yourself plenty of incentive to keep up the work of exercise, dieting and getting through your normal workday. Make your meals as delicious as possible, while keeping them nourishing and low in fat. Select a variety of different foods through the week and adjust your menus to the season. Don't eliminate all of your pleasures, just adjust them to be better for you.

A good meal is still an incentive, but it doesn't have to wreck my health.

A hungry man is not a free man.
—ADLAI STEVENSON

You can be obsessive about food whether you are eating a lot or a little. When you are starving yourself to get thin and still thinking about food constantly, you are as much in the grips of an illness as the person who can never put down the spoon.

Be moderate in your eating habits. Eat enough to satisfy your physical appetite. When you are consumed with hunger you are not free to concentrate on anything else.

How boring to focus on food all day. Instead, I will eat comfortably and put my mind to other things.

Never assume a responsibility you can't see through, and when you refuse, be firm. It saves trouble for everyone. —DAVID SEABURY

When someone asks you to do something you don't want to do, just say, "No, thank you" (unless of course it's a work situation where you absolutely have no choice). You don't even owe them an explanation.

When our self-esteem is low we're so flattered that anyone would choose us that we agree to do things that offer us nothing in return. But our time is worth more than that. We need to save our efforts for the projects we care about so that we will be able to give them our best. We don't do people any favors when we take away the opportunity for them to find someone who's truly right for the job.

I don't have to be everyone's savior. I will give when I truly have something to offer.

OCTOBER 29

They say butter is gold in the morning, silver at noon, but it is lead at night.
— JONATHAN SWIFT

Butter has gotten a bad rap in recent years. Packing more than twelve grams of fat and one hundred and eight calories into every tablespoon, it definitely needs to be approached with caution.

If it's a food you love and don't want to give up completely, eat it in dishes where you get the most possible enjoyment. Be selective. If you love butter's natural flavor, eliminate it from your cooking and just eat it occasionally on good bread—being careful how thick you spread it. If you can't resist a butter-based sauce now and then, indulge only on special occasions and give yourself just a small portion, sending the leftovers home with someone else so you won't be tempted to do a midnight refrigerator raid.

I may not be able to eliminate my dietary cravings, but I can manage them if I use care.

OCTOBER 30

Man's mettle is tested both in adversity and in success. — MADAME CHIANG KAI-SHEK

Learn to appreciate and absorb the full spectrum of experience that is available to you. A long-term program such as this allows you to build up the strength you will need to deal with any challenge that comes your way. Welcome troublesome times as opportunities to test your mettle and increase your confidence. Enjoy your successes as well and learn to handle them gracefully. This is not a race to reach your goal weight; it is a program you will learn to live by.

Every experience plays a role in my growth.

Since hunger is the most primitive and permanent of human wants, men always eat, but since their wish not to be a mere animal is also profound, they have always attended with special care to the manners which conceal the fact that at the table we are animals feeding.

—JOHN ERSKINE

Do you typically "wolf" down your meals? Do you "pig" out when you are alone?

Pay attention today not only to *what* you eat, but *how* you eat. Consider dressing for dinner, in the old-fashioned sense of putting on a clean outfit and freshening your hair and face. Put together an attractive table arrangement or at least clear a nice spot for yourself wherever you eat. Chew slowly and really taste the food. Put some effort into the conversation if you're eating with others, not just settling for the same topics you always discuss. And when you're finished with the meal, clear the dishes and relax for a few minutes before you rush off to your next activity.

Eating in a "civilized" manner can add to the enjoyment of the meal.

NOVEMBER 1

There are days when it seems impossible to be thrilled by anything, when a perverse dreariness holds the mind; and then all of a sudden the gentle and wistful mood flows back, and the world is full of beauty to the brim.

—A. C. BENSON

Our moods change continually. If we pay attention, we can see they are linked, one to another, in a kind of circular pattern. This ring of emotions, like a mandala, revolves inside us: melancholy, rage, happiness, fear, calm, contentment, anxiety.

Sometimes emotions are aroused by events in our lives, and sometimes they seem to have a life of their own. We can learn from them, but we don't have to be slaves to them. They are part of the landscape that we can step back from and view from a distance. Sometimes we see things more clearly when we're farther away.

I can patiently wait out one emotion because I know another will soon appear.

You can travel fifty thousand miles in America without once tasting a piece of good bread.
— HENRY MILLER

In seeking convenience, a long shelf life, and economy in our food, we have unfortunately sacrificed flavor. In the bread section of our local supermarket, for example, we may have fifty or more varieties from which to choose. But honestly, do any of them really taste good compared to fresh-baked bread from your own kitchen or a top-notch bakery? No, many taste vaguely like sawdust or cardboard, with a texture that's not much better. Other supermarket foods—some of the packaged and canned products for example—are even worse.

But few of us have time to cook everything from scratch, so what can we do? We can search out prepared foods of higher quality, possibly from small local businesses that aren't concerned with creating products that have a five-year shelf life. We can also find shortcuts in our cooking so that preparing a meal with fresh ingredients can be quick and easy.

I will search out true quality in the foods I eat.

NOVEMBER 3

Life is what happens to us while we are making other plans. —THOMAS LA MAANCE

We have this funny idea about life—it always seems to be "out there" somewhere caught in a Kodak moment. But on the contrary, it is in every single day that we eat and sleep and breathe. It is the night you stay up late with your little girl when she can't sleep. It is the dreadful blind date last week and the serendipitous, lovely day at the beach that made up for it.

Life isn't out there only when our ducks are lined up just right and our big plans can finally come to fruition; life is right here, right now.

Do I allow myself to appreciate that this is my life? If not, when will I start living?

NOVEMBER 4

Do what you can, with what you have, where you are. —THEODORE ROOSEVELT

During those periods when stress pops up in your life, it is sometimes difficult to deal with it and focus on weight reduction at the same time. But don't give up your good eating and exercise habits; just temporarily loosen your requirements a little if you need to. Stay as healthy as you can to help yourself through the hard times, but don't increase your stress level by placing unreasonable demands on yourself.

I will do what I can, even through difficult periods.

The best sauce in the world is hunger.
— CERVANTES

When we never allow ourselves to feel hunger, we deprive ourselves of the pleasure of truly appreciating a meal. Try an experiment today. Ignore the clocks and designated meal times and let your stomach tell you when to eat. Feel what it's like to get hungry and satisfy those pangs. Make your meals easily accessible so that you won't have to wait long once you're ready to eat.

If you're not hungry when everyone else around you is eating, resist the urge to go along with the group—nibble on a small salad instead. If you're going to a party and feel the need for something in your hand when you circulate, try a glass of club soda or plate of raw vegetables. What is this like? Do you really miss the food? Or do you feel better not eating than you would if you had eaten without hunger?

Today I will eat only when I'm hungry. This way I will learn my real need for food.

NOVEMBER 6

Vitality shows not only in the ability to persist but the ability to start over.
—F. SCOTT FITZGERALD

If a thin person eats too much of a meal do we say he is a glutton? No. We think of him as a thin person who ate too much on that occasion. Yet, when a person who is overweight does the same thing, he often uses it as proof to himself that he is a pig.

If you've been eating well most of the time, but slip up and have a bad day, don't start calling yourself names. Resist the temptation to go into the "I've always been fat, I always will be fat, I am a fat person" routine.

No one exists in a fixed state. Everything is changeable. Just because you ate like a glutton one day does not mean that you are one. Learn to separate your individual actions from who you are or can be.

One mistake does not cancel out all of my efforts.

NOVEMBER 7

We awaken in others the same attitude of mind we hold toward them. —ELBERT HUBBARD

Did you ever go out in a foul mood and find everyone else's behavior to be abominable? Did it seem that on this day especially, drivers were rude, pedestrians were out of line, and everyone in general seemed hostile? Do you think there is any connection between how you felt that day and how the world presented itself to you?

We give off powerful messages to others nonverbally. When they perceive us as hostile to them, they respond in kind (unless they're feeling unusually generous that day). Literally, what you give out is what you get back.

The Christian saying to treat others as I want to be treated makes sense practically and morally.

NOVEMBER 8

In all affairs, love, religion, politics, or business, it's a healthy idea, now and then, to hang a question mark on things you have long taken for granted. —BERTRAND RUSSELL

In past centuries, new ideas arrived at a snail's pace. But today our cult of information brings ideas to us at a dizzying rate. What we took to be truth a decade ago is now revealed as a fallacy. Shades of gray begin to appear where we once saw black and white.

It's healthy to keep an open mind, and healthy to examine our assumptions now and then. Many things you have taken for granted have been turned upside down. Give your beliefs a chance to catch up with the changes you've been going through in your daily life.

Nothing seems certain anymore, but I trust in my ability to navigate my way through the confusion.

NOVEMBER 9

It is the function of vice to keep virtue within reasonable bounds. —SAMUEL BUTLER

Guidelines for a behaviorial program are just that—guidelines. It's wise not to follow any plan too rigidly. Give yourself a little room to breathe now and then. Take it easy on the "shoulds" and don't kick yourself for every "could" that got away. So you could have done better—so what? You're not an automaton. Tolerate a little misbehavior in yourself now and then.

I want to avoid going to extremes.

Lettuce is like conversation: it must be fresh and crisp, and so sparkling that you scarcely notice the bitter in it. —C. D. WARNER

A meal is only as good as the ingredients that go into it. While some vegetables keep awhile—carrots and potatoes come to mind—others, such as lettuce, need to be picked and eaten quickly afterward. It makes such a difference in the taste and also influences the level of nutrition present in the food.

Adopt the old-fashioned custom of making small but frequent shopping trips for your produce. This discourages you from stocking up on vegetables that gradually lose their potency and flavor by week's end.

I will seek out the freshest of the fresh foods.

Spinach is the broom of the stomach.
—FRENCH PROVERB

Fruits and vegetables . . . fruits and vegetables. Make this a mantra that you repeat to yourself throughout the day. Chances are you don't get nearly enough of either one, especially vegetables—most people don't. The USDA recommends five servings a day. These are the life-giving foods; keep them in the forefront of your mind so they become the first thing you think of when you're hungry and seeking something to eat.

After a period of adjustment, you may notice your digestion improving (without artificial laxatives) as they clear out your stomach, and your energy level increasing as you lighten up.

Fruits and vegetables keep my digestive system on track. I'll get plenty every day to keep my body functioning properly.

If one says: I cannot come because that is my hour to be alone, one is considered rude, egotistical, or strange. What a commentary on our civilization, when being alone is considered suspect; when one has to apologize for it, make excuses, hiding the fact that one practices it — like a secret vice! —ANNE MORROW LINDBERGH

Time for yourself is not a luxury, it is something you must have. Everyone needs different amounts of time spent in solitude. You'll know if you're not getting enough of it, because you won't feel quite right when you don't.

When you take time for yourself, there's no need to offer an explanation to other people about how you spend it, whether it's lazing around in your pajamas on the weekend, catching up on some reading or caring for your plants. We don't even have to apologize to our spouses for taking a day off now and then to be by ourselves. This has nothing to do with them. No insult intended; we just need to recharge our batteries.

I cannot focus on myself when I'm taking care of everyone else. I need to set aside my own special time.

NOVEMBER 13

Even if it doesn't work, there is something healthy and invigorating about direct action.
—HENRY MILLER

When you're trying to resist the siren song of the sweet and salty junk-food products, one of the best things you can do is get out and get active. Remove yourself from the source of temptation. Try some new activities, look up old friends, jump into the swing of things. It may not be the ultimate reducing trick, but it's better than sitting at home thinking about what you're missing.

What activities are going on in my area right now that I might like to get involved in?

NOVEMBER 14

Strength is a matter of the made-up mind.
—JOHN BEECHER

If you've been radically uneven in your weight-loss program—dieting strictly, then slipping up; eating well, then eating junk—perhaps the problem lies in a lack of commitment.

As with all else in life, timing is everything in dieting. You may have a desire to lose weight, but lack the willingness to do the work. Or you may want to be slender, but part of you believes you aren't yet ready to slim down.

You must have a firm conviction that you can and should take this path. If it's not there, don't beat yourself up. Rather than attempting a huge weight loss under these conditions, just focus on eating well. When the time is right, you'll be ready to do the work.

Have I committed myself to weight loss and toning?

NOVEMBER 15

Extreme busyness, whether at school or college, work or market, is a symptom of deficient vitality; and a faculty for idleness implies a catholic appetite and a strong sense of personal identity.
— ROBERT LOUIS STEVENSON

It takes courage in our busy-busy world to admit to doing nothing. As much as we allow that we can't possibly "have it all," it's fashionable to try to anyway. Every morning the race begins anew.

We must make an effort to say no now and then and revitalize ourselves with purely idle endeavors. We have to reclaim our free time and decide how *we* want to use it—taking a nap, reading a book, writing in a journal or playing with our children. "Free" time should be just that, free, not scheduled with obligations, errands, and activities that fill every hour. Nor should we give in to the compulsion to drown out the quiet with television or other noisy machines.

My time is my own. How do I want to spend it?

NOVEMBER 16

What some call health, if purchased by perpetual anxiety about diet, isn't much better than tedious disease. — GEORGE DENNISON PRENTICE

One of the dangers of compulsive dieting is that we can become completely focused on our bodies and lose all perspective. It starts when dieting and exercising is all we think about or talk about or do. Mealtimes become an ordeal for our friends and family as we obsess about what we can and cannot eat. Outside interests fall by the wayside as we spend every free moment at the gym. At this point, we are out of control.

That's why it's so important to find balance in our lives. We must feed our minds so we have something else besides food to talk about. We need to pursue interests besides exercise so we will have something in our lives to care about when we get home from the gym.

Dieting is a means to an end, not a pursuit in and of itself.

Courage is fear holding on a minute longer.
—GENERAL GEORGE S. PATTON

The difference between eating and over-eating often lies in what you do with a single minute. It's the minute that you stop eating and remove yourself from the table before you start to overeat. It's the minute that you use to distract yourself when you feel a compulsion to binge and instead ride out the urge. It's also the minute that you give yourself to do one more lap, jog one more block, or hold that yoga position a little longer.

I can do anything for a minute. One minute is all it takes to do the right thing.

Choking will teach you to chew properly; falling will teach you to walk properly.
—MALAGASY PROVERB

It's an awful feeling to "bottom out" on a binge or some other part of the food-obsession cycle. You feel less than human when you've taken yourself to this place of little or no self-respect.

But just this experience, too, can be made fruitful. Sometimes we need to reach the bottom before we can begin our climb to the top. This is a dramatic lesson.

I may feel awful now, but I can do something positive with my pain.

To escape criticism—do nothing, say nothing, be nothing. —Elbert Hubbard

We are exposing ourselves to the world with our slimmer bodies. Do we want to expose our entire selves as well? The risk is criticism and rejection. The gain is an engagement with life that isn't possible when we hide away and play it safe. While we escape the criticism, we will also be losing out on the encouragement we might get.

I may find I garner a positive reception from others when I open myself up more.

It is well to remind ourselves that anxiety signifies a conflict, and so long as a conflict is going on, a constructive solution is possible.
—Rollo May

How hopeful this comment is. This means that even anxiety—seemingly useless—has a purpose. It can indictate to us that a conflict within us exists and that a solution may be found. If we could only turn our anxieties to these constructive ends, we would be fine. We must practice mindfulness to keep ourselves alert and aware. Only then can we see the action that is needed.

Emotions are like signposts directing me to decisions that need to be made. My desire helps bring my dreams to life.

A merry heart doeth good like a medicine.
—PROVERBS 17:22

There's more than one way to look at life's events. Try to approach life with a sense of humor instead of taking everything too seriously. As much as possible make it a point to "lighten up."

Learning to laugh at minor mishaps and everyday irritations instead of getting ourselves all worked up is so much better for our health. It improves the spirits of everyone around us and makes us a lot more pleasant to be around. And it improves the quality of our day too.

I can find the lighter side in most things.

Nothing is more sad than the death of an illusion. —ARTHUR KOESTLER

We have learned something new about ourselves by going through this journey. We are saying goodbye to our illusions. We can allow ourselves some time to feel sad about this. A feeling of loss should not be a surprise; goodbyes are always painful. We can spend a few quiet minutes today honoring the memories.

I will acknowledge my feelings of loss.

If Time, so fleeting, must, like humans, die, let it be filled with good food and good talk, and then embalmed in the perfumes of conviviality.
—M. F. K. FISHER

In many cultures, companionship is essential to the art of dining. The food is only part of the meal. The other vital element is the gathering of people together to break bread, share a meal, commune. Dinner—or lunch or breakfast—is a time to connect with others.

This may seem an impossible goal if you have demanding toddlers, teenagers always on the run, or a work schedule that doesn't allow time for sit-down meals. In that case, start small and be creative. Designate one meal a week—Sunday supper or a mid-week dinner—as a special family event that everyone will honor. Keep it casual and involve each person in the preparation of the meal. Ask everyone to bring a story to share or topic to discuss.

After the food is on the table, sit down and enjoy it. Take time to appreciate the abundance of good food, love, and companionship in your life.

I will make it a habit to count my blessings and not just my calories.

That a man should eat and drink and enjoy himself, in return for all his labours, is a gift of God. —ECCLESIASTES 3:13

The start of the holiday season brings days that will test your diet resolve. But there's nothing to fear if you approach the dinner meal sensibly. All you have to do is follow the same rules that you usually eat by, giving yourself a little more margin for error.

Make the bulk of your meal the vegetable, fruit, and grain dishes that contain little or no fat. Then dish up tastes of a few of your favorite "bad" holiday foods and skip the things you don't love. If there's going to be nothing you can eat at a party, bring a couple of low-fat dishes yourself.

And then give thanks for it all.

I can relax and enjoy the wonderful holiday meal to come.

Wine brings gaiety and high spirits, if a man knows when to drink and when to stop.
—ECCLESIASTICUS 31:28

Those who are watching their weight should also watch their alcoholic intake. Alcohol can be a contributor to weight problems: Alcohol contains mostly empty calories—sugar with no nutrition. The high sugar content can trigger binges in those who are sensitive to it. It slows down metabolism, and drinking goes hand in hand with overeating and encourages consumption of salty, high-fat snacks.

But if alcohol intake is truly within your ability to control, you can still enjoy a glass of wine with dinner or a drink now and then. Just don't allow it to become a bad habit.

I'm not going to allow alcohol to throw off the progress of my weight-loss program.

A man should always consider how much he has more than he wants, and how much more unhappy he might be than he really is.
—JOSEPH ADDISON

It's good to stop and count our blessings on a regular basis, giving thanks for all that is ours. Each of us possesses so much more than we know. To remind ourselves of at least a few of those things gives us a perspective on how lucky we really are. The next time we are feeling sorry for ourselves, we can think back and know we are better off than we feel at the moment.

I am blessed with more than I even need.

Better by far that you should forget and smile, than you should remember and be sad.
—CHRISTINA ROSSETTI

If you have very real memories of pain or sadness in your life, coming to terms with those experiences—perhaps with the help of a therapist—is probably a necessary step to moving beyond them. But once you have faced them, you don't necessarily have to remind yourself of them again and again every day. If you were extremely heavy during one period of your childhood, nothing says that you must keep pictures of yourself from that time around in your photo albums for every visitor to peruse. If there was a traumatic incident, you don't have to revisit it in your mind continually. Put it aside and step into the present. Concentrate on the joy you can have today.

I've had my share of pain. I don't need to dwell on it.

NOVEMBER 28

My soul is dark with stormy riot, directly traceable to diet. —SAMUEL HOFFENSTEIN

One of the unpleasant side effects of a bad diet is its negative effect on our mood and disposition.

Excessive amounts of sugar and caffeine can take us up and down on an emotional roller coaster. A diet made up entirely of junk food can leave us cranky and unsatisfied. Too much of any kind of food can put us in a state of lethargy, unwilling to do more than snooze and sit around.

So pay attention to how your diet affects your emotional health. Watch how foods alter your mood and keep track of those that stir up allergies. In the end, you should follow a diet that makes you feel good physically and emotionally.

Food can work like a drug on my moods. I will respect its power and use it wisely.

NOVEMBER 29

What does not destroy me, makes me strong. —FRIEDRICH NIETZSCHE

Every time we fail we get a little wiser. Each time we stumble we learn something about ourselves. We become stronger with each of our setbacks, not weaker. When we turn them around into a learning experience, they become positives, not negatives. I don't have to curse my mistakes any longer; they are my teachers.

I grow stronger in my determination every day.

Enthusiasm is the best protection in any situation. Wholeheartedness is contagious. Give yourself, if you wish to get others.
—DAVID SEABURY

Now is your time to shine! Cultivate enthusiasm in your life, and it will attract people who are enthusiastic about you. Step out and say who you are and what you believe. Give the parts of yourself you never thought you'd share. Let the goodness that is inside you emerge. You have so much to offer and you've hidden yourself away for so long.

I can dance, dream, sing, and my life will be all the richer for it.

DECEMBER 1

If you have formed the habit of checking on every new diet that comes along, you will find that, mercifully, they all blur together, leaving you with only one definite piece of information: French fried potatoes are out.
—JEAN KERR

Check the national best-seller lists and you'll find a diet book or two gracing the charts at any given time. Some of them make a lot of sense and even add something to the growing body of nutritional literature. Most, however, are no more than junk food for the mind.

Avoid diets that advocate eating only one or two foods to lose weight and those that cut out entire food groups, such as fruits, vegetables, proteins, or grains. Stay away from diets that reduce your intake to less than one thousand calories a day. Rigid diets that give you prescribed eating plans may help you lose weight, but will not be so helpful in teaching you to keep it off once you go back to your normal eating habits. On the other hand, diets that teach you how to prepare easy meals using low-fat, minimally processed foods can be helpful.

You're not in this to lose weight for six months and then gain it back, so look for those diets that provide long-term guidelines for eating right.

I will resist the lure of the unhealthy, quick-weight-loss plans.

DECEMBER 2

One should want only one thing and want it constantly. Then one is sure of getting it. But I desire everything and consequently get nothing. Each time I discover, and too late, that one thing had come to me while I was running after another. —ANDRÉ GIDE

While you're in the midst of changing your eating and exercise habits, go easy on yourself in the rest of your life. There is some stress involved in making these alterations, so don't make the task more difficult by stretching your emotional resources over too wide a field. Even if your tendency is to aim for high goals in all areas of your life, learn to prioritize and put your health program at the top. Go slowly with the others until this goal is well on its way to completion.

Easy does it: one step at a time.

DECEMBER 3

Experience teaches only the teachable.
—ALDOUS HUXLEY

Everything in life can teach us something —if we allow ourselves to learn something new. If not, we go on endlessly repeating old patterns—running hard, but never moving forward. What a colossal waste of time that is.

I can learn much if I keep my mind open.

DECEMBER 4

To love, and to be hurt often, and to love again — this is the brave and happy life.
— J. E. BUCKROSE

Food may have seemed like your friend in the past, but it is not really serving you today if it prevents you from getting what you really want and need, which is love.

Slowly, venture out of the house, out of your shell, and experiment with bringing new people into your life. Give something of yourself. Share a private thought. Take a chance with a new friend.

You'll encounter some painful experiences and enjoy others that are truly fulfilling. Both are more satisfying than settling for a poor substitute for love.

Love is what I really want. I must go out and get it.

DECEMBER 5

Bitterness imprisons life; love releases it. Bitterness paralyzes life; love empowers it. Bitterness sours life; love sweetens it. Bitterness sickens life; love heals it. Bitterness blinds life; love anoints its eye. — HARRY EMERSON FOSDICK

No matter how many awful events come our way, we do not have to become bitter. Letting ourselves descend into bitterness means we have given up on ourselves — thrown in the towel. We have, in essence, proclaimed, "Life is bad and will continue to be so."

Bitterness goes against logic in its refusal to see that good things do happen to us, too. We close our eyes to half of the experiences life offers. But we should remember that even a gambler's losing streak turns around eventually if he stays at the table long enough.

Opening my heart to love can heal the pain.

Total abstinence is easier than perfect moderation. —St. Augustine

Some nutrition experts now say it is easier to switch over to nonfat products completely than it is to go halfway by eating those that contain some fat. The same is true with sugar, alcohol, and meat; you may be more successful cutting them out altogether than in trying to moderate your intake.

There are a number of reasons for this. One is that it's simpler to be given black-and-white choices than to have to determine how much is too much. Another is that you will lose your taste for the substance if you avoid it completely, rather than torturing yourself by sampling it in small amounts. And, in the case of fat, when you cut it out you will usually drop weight faster than if you just moderate your intake of it, so you get your diet rewards sooner, and that makes it easier to keep going.

Would changing my diet more radically work better for me?

DECEMBER 7

It is a funny thing about life — if you refuse to accept anything but the best you very often get it.
— W. SOMERSET MAUGHAM

As we improve our diet and begin to seek quality in everything we eat, we may find this rubbing off on other aspects of our lives. Treatment we would have settled for in the past no longer seems acceptable. Instead of making do with products that are second-best we wait until we can find what we really want. As we learn to respect our bodies more, it becomes natural to do the same thing in the rest of our lives.

I will seek quality in everything I eat and everything I do.

DECEMBER 8

Gluttony slays more than the sword.
— ENGLISH PROVERB

A perfect figure or a toned physique may strike some as being a luxury, not a necessity, and so they toy half-heartedly with diet after diet. But put those same people in the hospital with a heart attack and watch them change their bad eating and drinking habits! Don't wait until obesity takes its toll on your health. Do something about it now, while you are still in good condition. Don't abuse your body with food and drink. Eat to maintain your best health.

There are serious health consequences to poor eating habits.

I got the blues thinking of the future, so I left off and made some marmalade. It's amazing how it cheers one up to shred oranges or scrub the floor.
— D. H. LAWRENCE

Thinking about a day in the future when we're thirty pounds lighter can sometimes give us hope, and at other times fill us with desperation. Will we ever get there? How will we get there? What will we do when we arrive?

At such times it's better to leave off with the worrying and plant ourselves back in the present moment. Getting involved in a physical task that requires our attention can give us a blessed respite from the mental gymnastics. Shredding oranges, scrubbing the floor, washing the dishes, or mowing the lawn: These are simple tasks that require no decision making or analysis, yet improve our life in a small way. Constructive action saves the day again.

I can chase away worries about the future by concentrating on improving my life in little ways today.

DECEMBER 10

Every man in the world is better than someone else. And not as good as someone else.
—WILLIAM SAROYAN

Some people have a quality or trait that you admire. Maybe you even envy them a little for it. But let it stop there. When you seek what someone else has because it looks good on them, you're chasing after an elusive rainbow. You've devalued yourself, overlooking who you are, what you have to offer, and where you should be going. You trample over your own dreams in the quest to reach theirs.

We each have our talents and our own destiny.

DECEMBER 11

The future comes one day at a time.
—DEAN ACHESON

It's not possible to go too far in reminding ourselves to take things one day at a time. We're so used to jumping ahead and living in the future, and when we do that we can overwhelm ourselves with worries about what might happen. But we can't *really* live in the future; this moment is the only thing we have. We can only act now to build our futures. It's easier than we think.

Dramatic change seems overwhelming, but when I take it day by day it becomes manageable.

DECEMBER 12

I have had many periods of wretchedness, but with energy and, above all, with illusions, I pulled through them all.

—HONORÉ DE BALZAC

Be your own best dieting friend. Tell yourself the things you need to hear to go on with your program. Leave little notes around the house for yourself, congratulating you on your progress and urging you on. Put energy into this diet endeavor. You are not going to stop and give up, so you might as well make the effort as pleasurable as possible.

I will be creative in finding ways to keep myself motivated through difficult times.

DECEMBER 13

All the great speakers were bad speakers first.

—RALPH WALDO EMERSON

As you learn the best way for you to eat and exercise, keep in mind that this is a process, not something you should have mastered on the first day. You've had a lot of practice doing things the wrong way, so give yourself some time to learn to do it right. No one is born knowing how to do everything perfectly. We all need to make mistakes and learn from them. Suffering through being bad at something is the only way to become great later on.

The point is to practice and learn how to do it.

DECEMBER 14

The world owes all its onward impulses to men ill at ease. The happy man inevitably confines himself within ancient limits.

—NATHANIEL HAWTHORNE

You've been prompted on this journey by the restlessness in your heart. It's not been easy to rearrange your life and change your habits, but you have done it. And you could have done nothing at all. Give yourself some credit. And it all goes back to the day when you felt so awful inside, troubled by the state of things in your life. That miserable day played an important role in your life!

Restlessness and anxiety can be important catalysts for change.

DECEMBER 15

At any given moment, life is completely senseless. But viewed over a period, it seems to reveal itself as an organism existing in time, having a purpose, tending in a certain direction.

—ALDOUS HUXLEY

It's easy for us to feel adrift at times. We go from one activity to another and then start over again. Events appear to be unrelated, meaningless. As we get older though, we do see a pattern. A sense of purpose begins to appear, one we could never have recognized at the time. It's as though some unseen hand is coaxing us like a strand of yarn into a specfic place on a loom. We can't see the design from where we are, but we can trust that one will appear.

My life may have a purpose of which I am not yet aware.

DECEMBER 16

In this age, which believes that there is a shortcut to everything, the greatest lesson to be learned is that the most difficult way is, in the long run, the easiest. —HENRY MILLER

We do everything we can to avoid facing our inner demons. We put off seeking therapy. We put a happy face on everything even though something inside us knows better. We keep the lights on at night so we never have to confront ourselves in the dark. And we run.

But in fleeing the difficult lesson, we find ourselves tripping and taking painful falls because we're running in desperation and can't see where we're going.

We create more pain for ourselves than if we turned and looked at the truth we are trying to avoid. In running from our fears we stand in the way of our own healing.

With a deep breath I will turn my attention inside.

DECEMBER 17

Chance is always powerful. Let your hook be always cast. In the pool where you least expect it, will be a fish. —OVID

We increase our chances of finding good luck when we prepare for it. We don't have to watch for it restlessly, we only need to be ready for it when it appears.

We know that something new and different is on its way. When it arrives we can be happy, for we now know how to take care of ourselves. And thus, others will take good care of us, too.

I am learning to expect the unexpected.

DECEMBER 18

Do not protect yourself by a fence, but rather by your friends. —CZECH PROVERB

There's no substitute for a good friend. As you strip away the layers of fat protection you have built up as a physical barrier from others, you learn who you can trust to let in closer. These are the people who will help defend you when the world closes in. Build friendships and extended family to protect yourself from isolation. Humans are social animals; when we are alone, we are vulnerable. When we have companionship, we benefit from the strength of the group.

As I lay my fences down, I allow my good friends in.

DECEMBER 19

Better one hand full and peace of mind, than both fists full and toil that is chasing the wind.
—ECCLESIASTES 4.6

Those who spend all of their time exercising and dieting—and no time healing their emotional, spiritual, and mental wounds—are setting themselves up for difficulties down the line. The person who takes the dieting more slowly but spends time cultivating better mental patterns is light years ahead of the game. Without peace of mind, a thin person risks the curse of anorexia. No matter how slender an anorexic gets, her mind is never convinced she is thin enough. However, the person who has healed her mind is at peace with herself whether she's at her ideal weight or heavier.

Peace of mind means we accept ourselves no matter what our condition.

DECEMBER 20

Enough is as good as a feast.
—JOHN HEYWOOD

Many restaurants serve enormous portions of food—much more than any of us should reasonably eat at one time. But just because you are served a family-sized plate of spaghetti and a half loaf of garlic toast does not mean you have to eat it all. Halfway through the meal, pause for a few moments and ask yourself if you are still hungry. Pace yourself from that point on, keeping tabs on your feeling of fullness. Stop eating when you are no longer hungry, no matter how much food is left on the plate.

How many times have you continued eating past this point and regretted it later that night or the next morning? Don't do that to yourself this time.

If I'm not hungry, I don't need to finish the meal.

DECEMBER 21

A single event can awaken within us a stranger totally unknown to us. To live is to be slowly born. —ANTOINE DE SAINT EXUPÉRY

There are layers to us, aspects of our personalities of which we are not even aware. Change is a process of alchemy—different elements reacting against each other in unpredictable ways. Part of the beauty of living is to follow this unwinding mystery that is our lives. We unfold and open ourselves to new experiences as life goes on.

Who knows what event might change my life forever?

DECEMBER 22

We receive love—from our children as well as others—not in proportion to our demands or sacrifices or needs, but roughly in proportion to our own capacity to love. —ROLLO MAY

Many of us feel we deserve love from certain people in our lives—our children, parents, siblings, spouses. When we don't get it, we feel cheated. Some of us react by trying to demand love as our birthright—an approach that rarely works. Others withdraw, afraid to express their disappointment.

The solution lies in learning to give love, without requirements or expectations, to everyone you can. As your capacity for loving grows, so does your ability to receive it.

The more we chase after love, the more it eludes us.

DECEMBER 23

That best portion of a good man's life, his little, nameless, unremembered acts of kindness and love. —WILLIAM WORDSWORTH

In lieu of creating a grand work of timeless art today, there's something else you can do to give your life some purpose or meaning. Perform a small kindness—something quiet. Look for ways to improve a person's life—even if only for the moment—but choose acts that don't call attention to themselves. Keep it to yourself as your private pleasure. The good feeling you get from these little kindnesses will be like stored firewood that keeps you warm on cold nights.

There are so many ways I can be kind to other people without going out of my way.

Congealed fat is pretty much the same, irrespective of the delicacy around which it is congealed.
—CLEMENT FREUD

To release ourselves from the grips of our cravings, we may need to look at them in a clear light. What are those tasty treats we pine for really made of? More than likely, animal fat. So many of the foods we are drawn to so powerfully contain it. Animal fat is what makes the bacon crispy, the pie crust flaky, and the foie gras rich and smooth.

Find a way to deromanticize these foods. If it is a dish usually served warm, chill it overnight and look at the amount of fat congealed on the plate the next morning. Or if you usually buy a dish already prepared, fix it yourself, to see how much fat it really contains.

You don't need to lose all pleasure from the dish, but you do want to see it for what it is. When you eat it next time, you'll know what you're getting into and may choose a smaller portion.

My body may respond instinctively to high-fat foods, but I don't have to blindly consume them.

DECEMBER 25

I sometimes think we expect too much of Christmas Day. We try to crowd into it the long arrears of kindliness and humanity of the whole year. —DAVID GRAYSON

Christmas and Thanksgiving deserve their reputations as the two days dieters fear most. Certainly they can be happy occasions. But the combination of high expectations, family tensions, a table full of rich foods, and societal license to stuff yourself on these days can mean disaster for dieters.

You can take some of the pressure off yourself today by lowering your expectations. Remember, it's a day like any other. You don't have to be the perfect daughter or son or parent today. There's no need to show a perfect face or bottle up everything you feel. Go easy—on yourself and everyone else. If you find yourself overeating in response to emotional discomfort, stop and look for an alternative: Step outside for some fresh air or strike up a conversation with your favorite aunt or grandson.

I won't expect perfection today. I will accept myself and others as we are.

DECEMBER 26

The important thing is not what they think of me, it is what I think of them.
—QUEEN VICTORIA

Get off the "What do they think of me?" roller coaster. Worrying about what other people think of you and basing your valuation of yourself on their judgment is giving them more power than they deserve.

They might not even be people whom you like or respect. Once you've determined that this is so, don't even waste too much time pondering "What do I think of them?" The important question is "What do I think of myself?"

Other people's opinions of me may be based on things that have nothing to do with me. I can ignore them.

DECEMBER 27

The highest reward for a man's toil is not what he gets for it but what he becomes of it.
—JOHN RUSKIN

You've been paying a great deal of attention to the care of your own body and improving the way you look. Be sure to give some thought to the other, less tangible, areas in your life. Balance the extra time you give to yourself by remembering to care about other people too.

Uncover your purpose for living so that you aren't disappointed after you've lost the extra weight. Give yourself a reason to be proud of yourself beyond the inches you have shed. Your weight-loss program would be a disaster if you dropped all the pounds you wanted to lose but ended up miserable and mean.

A beautiful body is an empty vessel without a beautiful spirit inside.

If men could regard the events of their own lives with more open minds, they would frequently discover that they did not really desire the things they failed to obtain. —ANDRÉ MAUROIS

When we look back at our failed attempts at dieting in the past, we should also contemplate what else was going on in our lives at the time. Were we under a lot of stress, or maybe going through a painful emotional period? Were we hanging onto a food obsession as one of the few acceptable comforts we had? Were we, despite lip service to the contrary, not really willing to let go of our bad food habits at the time? Was our extra weight serving a purpose for us?

Understanding our own histories can help us today when we are wondering how we could have failed at our dieting so many times before. The truth is, we can't say we failed if we weren't really committed to losing weight in the first place.

If I look closely at my "failures" I may find an explanation for them.

DECEMBER 29

When one door of happiness closes, another opens; but often we look so long at the closed door that we do not see the one which has been opened for us. —HELEN KELLER

You are shedding a familiar habit that has served you well in the past. Say goodbye and watch as it goes away. Then mourn it until you miss it no more.

Now the real fun begins. Keep your eyes open to the new possibilities that will eventually present themselves to you. Even if you can't see what lies in the future, you know that something new will come to take the place of old ways. Pay attention so you can recognize it when it appears.

I will be cared for. Everything is going to be all right.

DECEMBER 30

The world is all gates, all opportunities, strings of tension waiting to be struck.
—RALPH WALDO EMERSON

So many new experiences await you now. When you have removed the barriers to living fully and joyously, you see how many doors suddenly open to you. Take your time exploring them; you don't have to walk through them all. Take care of yourself at this time more than ever. In a way, you're like a young child. Don't overwhelm yourself with choices and challenges.

My life has a new richness.

Good habits are not made on birthdays, nor Christian character at the new year. The workshop of character is everyday life. The uneventful and commonplace hour is where the battle is lost or won. —MALTBIE D. BABCOCK

Another year is gone, and a new year is on the horizon. Perhaps it has occurred to you that your battle with weight is not yet over. You did better this year than you did during the holidays last year, but still didn't entirely escape the temptation of overeating. So what do you do to shed those extra pounds? Here's where the real challenge begins.

Resist the urge to try to lose the extra pounds fast by starving yourself after the New Year as you might have done in the past. Instead, resume your healthy weight-loss program: Go back to eating low-fat, low-sugar foods, getting regular exercise, and taking care of your mental, spiritual, and emotional health.

It will take longer to lose the extra weight this way, but it will stay off longer. In the meantime, you will reinforce the good habits that will keep you healthy the rest of your life.

Weight management is a lifetime endeavor. I can take it slowly.

About the Author

ANNE COLBY writes about health, nutrition, and other lifestyle topics for such publications as *Bon Appetit*, *Modern Maturity*, *Woman's Day*, the *Los Angeles Times*, *Sunset*, *Los Angeles*, and *LACMA Physician*. She has edited a food-marketing newsletter and is a former editor of *Home* magazine. She is currently a staff editor at the *Los Angeles Times*.